How to Talk to Your Aspie

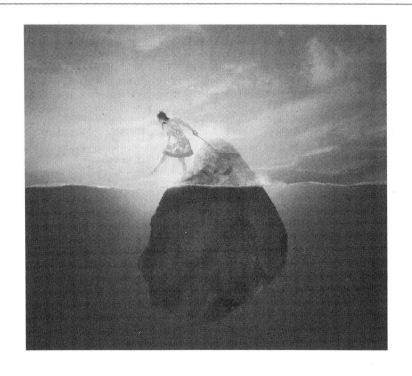

Amanda J Harrington

Contents

7

Introduction

I wish I could talk to people, you know? Talk to them in the same way as when I write my blog or my books. The written word comes so easily compared to the stilted, stuttering, compacted conversations I offer in the real world. How does this happen? Why can I write it and not say it? It is the same brain behind both things!

And this is how I came to the second book in my Crazy Girl in an Aspie World series. I realised that a disproportionate amount of my blog posts were spent analysing communication and explaining how hard it can be for aspies to talk to other people, let alone explain their feelings.

People who found my blog searched using phrases like, 'talk to an aspie', 'why can't aspies talk,' 'weird aspie talk' and 'strange things that aspies say'. Yes, we are weird and say strange things or we can't talk or people try to talk to us and come away confused.

Faced with the real world, lots of aspies freeze and need to give themselves a push to carry on into the maelstrom. It is hard out there. The world is filled with a myriad of aggravating events which impact on the aspie psyche and leave us reeling as if in pain. On top of all this, we are expected to communicate too.

I often think that communicating with other people is like trying to talk in the middle of a thunder storm or while being chased by wild, hungry animals: the other person doesn't see the storm or the pursuit, they only see *you*, stood like a great wedge of cheese, staring at them with your face fixed in confused thought. They wonder why you don't speak, they ask if anything is wrong and then they leave.

The storm abates, the animals vanish and the aspie is left alone, quiet, annoyed with their inability to communicate but at the same time relieved that the danger is over. They can relax until the next time someone wants something from them. And maybe by then they will have got the hang of this talking business.

This book is titled, 'How to Talk to Your Aspie' but much of it is written from the aspie viewpoint. Some of these chapters are adapted from my popular blog, Crazy Girl in an Aspie World and are included because other people have found them relevant and helpful.

Family, friends, best beloveds, have a look at the world from an aspie point of view and see how creative, frightening, annoying and enlightening it can be.

Amanda J Harrington

July 19th, 2014

http://aspie-girl.blogspot.co.uk/

1: Talking About Feelings

Can there be anything more like pulling teeth than talking about your feelings? Articulating how you feel and why you feel and how this makes you feel is so *difficult*! It often seems much better to avoid the conversation until another time and hope that somewhere between now and then, the whole feelings issue will have magically resolved itself so there is no need to talk about it after all.

Meltdowns are feelings in motion but they don't have to be explained. Actually talking about feelings is a way of expressing yourself which means opening a door wide to the outside world. No matter that the person on the other side of the door might be your best beloved: behind them stands the world, waiting for the chance to pour in and bring chaos to your carefully ordered inner self.

Feelings are tricky and uncontrollable, they make life awkward, they make you wonder if anything will ever be manageable. When feelings take over, you become a mess, a creature of instincts who cannot respond with wonderful, soothing logic. Feelings are there to trip you up and must be watched carefully. Talking about them means we have to let others watch them too. No wonder they hurt.

This section is all about feelings and the various ways aspies talk or avoid talking about them. It is not exhaustive – there are as many ways to avoid talking about feelings as there are aspies. And sometimes aspies *can* express their emotions but then can't listen and process the emotions of those closest to them.

Read on and know that you are not alone in sighing as your aspie vanishes over the horizon, hand raised in good bye and speed increasing as you call out, 'but I wanted to ask how you felt...'

How do you feel?

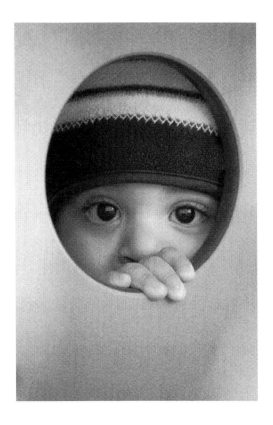

Your aspie is very good at explaining things in great detail, down to the toe caps worn by a character in an out-of-print novel by a French author in the 1920s. If you were listening, you could repeat the details of Theo the Philanderer to anyone not quick enough to get away. Also, your aspie can spell out exactly how they felt when they were queue-jumped in the local shop, including how many times it had happened, why it always happened to them (why did it always happen to them?) why that woman did what she did and why the checkout operator pretended it never happened.

So why is it when you want to know how your aspie feels about something close to your heart, or important to their life and wellbeing, they clam up and can barely remember their own name?

It's not too difficult, is it? Given the amount of detail forthcoming in so many other conversations, the appalled silence which greets you when you *ask* for information can make you feel a little indignant. It's not as if you don't know how to talk to your aspie and draw them out, is it? All these years of dealing with your own version of a wild goat with Wi-Fi should have prepared you for those rare occasions when you try to find their real and true feelings.

Except it doesn't work that way.

Winkling out the facts about the queue jumper can be bad enough: this is when your goat-steering skills are most often needed, for those times when you want to know actual details from real life. One question leads to another and then you steer the conversation back to the original question, coming at it from a new direction. It is all very familiar.

Eventually, you will realise your aspie was in the wrong queue or had forgotten they were waiting and left a gap big enough for people to think they weren't even in the queue or, more likely, were being taken advantage of by wily old ladies who know how to queue jump.

You come away with the hard-won details, probably wondering why it's so difficult to get a straight answer to a simple question. Next time you'll know better.

Except what if the next time isn't about queue jumping but concerns the innermost aspie? It could be the state of your relationship (ye gods! Good luck there!), how your aspie feels about school/college/work, how they feel about the new baby in the house or their elderly parent emigrating with a new partner.

Whatever important feelings are in sight, you want to know how your aspie is doing and as they don't often open up without prompting, you decide to ask…

Let me put it this way – describing old lady queue jumpers can be rather fun, even from the middle of an indignant rage. The clues are all there, the memory is fresh and even if the questions seem a little random or badly-phrased, your aspie will do their best to answer them.

But compare that to talking about *feelings*? And worse, being asked about them? Feelings, so elusive yet powerful, which simultaneously hide behind a metaphorical rock while driving you down into the mountain pass? How on earth is a person meant to explain those?

Feelings are all very well, but even if your aspie could explain them, why should they? Feelings get in the way of every single thing! They make life difficult, they make you do things you don't want to or get you upset when you can't do something. They are a big pig in the middle of the road and there is no ignoring them. The last thing aspies want to do is have to talk about them too.

Cue a wailing sound and flailing of arms as your aspie runs from the room. The slamming of a distant door tells you that Feelings will not be discussed today.

So other than employing hypnotism or a Vulcan mind meld, how do you find out about an aspie's feelings? Assuming you want more than a one-word answer, or the flailing of arms, you need to tread very carefully.

Be aware of how you have handled this kind of conversation in the past. Most likely, you can remember the times it didn't work, so make sure not to repeat your mistakes. Those conversations ending in drama or sulking are not the ones you want to relive.

For instance, my big fault when trying to talk to my aspie son is to fill in the blanks. If I ask him a question and there is a big gap, I jump in the gap and fill it with choices. Multiple-choice feelings, what could be better?! Usually it gets on his nerves to such an extent that he gives in and answers my original question just to shut me up. (I'm not advocating this as an approach that works because I only get a simple answer, not an in-depth explanation of how he is).

Think carefully about *why* you need to know something. For instance, if you want to know how your aspie feels about their mother getting married again, do you want to know how they feel because it's a big event or are you worried about them? If you simply want to talk about a parent's remarriage, you might find yourself chatting to the dog again. If your aspie doesn't see any great need to talk about their feelings, then they likely won't. But if you are worried about your aspie and sense they are fretting over the remarriage, it is probably a good idea to have the talk.

What I advise is making your reasons clear. Do not try to be chatty and jolly, leading up to the big talk about feelings. Aspies are not daft, you know. How many people do you think have tried to jolly them into things over the years? And then *you* try it, their best beloved! Do you think the goat doesn't know it's going to be tied up just because you hide the rope behind your back? Did no one else try to fool it that way?

Be honest and upfront. You need to state that you are worried and say *why* you are worried. Express your need to talk about how your aspie is feeling and leave bigger gaps than I do while you are waiting for them to respond.

If it is just a matter of your aspie talking about their feelings, then they probably won't do it, but if they think you are worried or upset for them and need to talk about it, you have more chance. Not a sure thing, you understand, but more likely.

And don't forget that today's failed conversation and energetic escape to the safe place of bedroom/bathroom/car/garden shed can be tomorrow's heart to heart. Yes, this is what works best, for me at least. A conversational firework started today might just need time to settle. Give it a while, a few hours or even a few days, and you might find that it has been looked at enough for them to come back to you and answer your questions.

This is the time when you succeed, those rare occasions when your aspie tells you what you need to know and what they need to express. Value it and cherish it, knowing it is a special event. Also, do not, whatever you do, take it as permission for other conversations along the same lines. Just because you had your feelings out today does not mean they can come out every day – access is granted as and when required so don't overuse it. And remember to close the door behind you.

How do I feel?

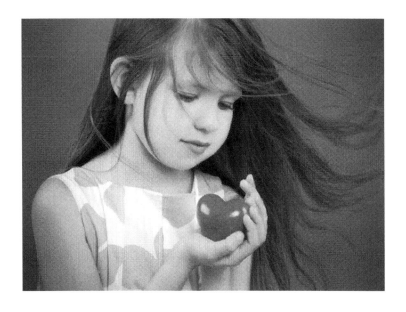

Communication is difficult enough but my heart never sinks faster than when someone wants to discuss my feelings. Many a useful conversation has fallen apart because I have felt like I am under the microscope, there to be examined and finally understood as my inner feelings are dissected and drawn out under the spotlight.

It really does feel this painful. I want people to like me and to understand me; I want to be proper friends and know what it is like to be able to turn to one another in times of trouble. I am a real human being with a full set of emotions and I don't mind feeling them. What I do mind is sharing them with other people.

To be probed, sorry, to be *asked how I feel*, is like an intrusion. One small question about my inner heart and I expect to be revealed to the whole world. It doesn't matter if I am asked by my family or a complete stranger, the panic surging through me is the same.

And the reason for this reaction? Perhaps it is rooted in all those times as a child when you are just starting to realise how complicated the world might be and then people turn to you and demand to know why you did such a thing, or what you think, or how you are. These simple requests, friendly or otherwise, are terrifying to small, uncertain children who have no idea about themselves, let alone anything else.

That feeling of being confronted by others, held accountable as if you understand your own behaviour and motivations, it stays with you into adulthood. You become adept at either sidestepping discussions on how you feel or offering whatever you think is an acceptable answer.

Turn it around and you have the reason why I don't ask you how *you* are feeling. I care about you, I hope you are happy, oh but please don't tell me how you feel. Don't involve me in your deepest, saddest, loneliest and loveliest of emotions. It is too much and it scares me rigid.

If I ask how you are, I would be glad to know you are well, that you haven't dropped anything heavy on your foot, that you continue to exist in a reasonably successful state. If you have practical problems, do share and I'm sure I can offer a wealth of solutions.

If your heart is broken though, I will fully console and hold your troubles within my hand: I just won't say anything that gives this away. I will hope your inner hurt heals and your smile lifts again. I will look in your face each time we meet to see if your eyes are brighter and your face less burdened. And then I will talk about the weather, all the while studying you to see if you are all right.

I am sorry my hand doesn't find its way into yours. I regret I rarely open the doors between us and that I peek through the spyhole instead. I wish, sometimes, I could be a different person who tells you how much I love you and wish good things for you.

We turn together and I tell you about the funny programme I watched last night, or a silly story I read online and I hope, in this small, unmatterful way, I can make you smile while you are with me.

Aspies make dull conversationalists

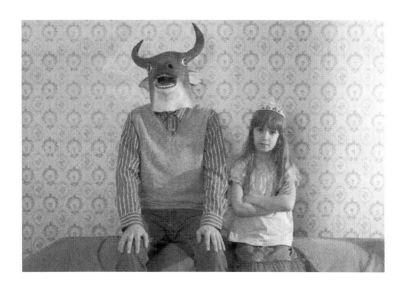

When you feel an emotion, you generally know how it affects you. Happiness is positive and makes you feel good, sadness is negative and makes you feel bad - nice and simple, like those smiley-face emoticons I'm meant to find so confusing.

Then you have the mixture of feelings which come as part of the human-bean package. It's no good expecting to have a standard set of emotions which are easily identified; as a human race we are programmed to be complex. If we weren't complex, there would be no reality TV shows. If we were straightforward, we would either smile when we greeted one another or whallop the other person and then smile.

Instead, we are plagued by a mess of feelings such as supposed pleasure at your friend coming to visit, followed by mortification that you forgot to shave your legs and are wearing shorts, then embarrassment that the cat finally got rid of last night's supper, irritation at your friend's tales of glory and, finally, blessed (but guilty) relief when the visit is over.

Afterwards, if someone asked me how the visit went I would say it was fine or okay and then relay any important news. I wouldn't dissect my feelings, I would just be left with the sense that visits are often stressful.

Feelings, good, bad, muddy or kaleidoscopic; they are a massive distraction when it comes to getting on with life. The friend's visit would be much more pleasant if I could stick with one emotion (even a less than positive one) and work around it. Start adding situations to emotions and you have a small panic building.

Throw in conversations which I am expected to enjoy and the feelings become a flying swarm all around me, biting at my face, zooming before my eyes, buzzing in my ears and dashing away as soon as I raise my hand to swat them.

The words in the conversation are complex enough when you can't quite see past the feelings but then you have to contribute and make sense and, on top of all of this, readers, take an interest in what the other person is saying!

You see, if I was feeling blank, or dull, or even sad, the emotions would be static and I could cope with the conversation. While I may not be any more interested, I would have more opportunity to pretend interest.

(I'm sorry if this sounds harsh. I am often interested in what people are saying, just not always the people I am meant to be listening to).

I have had countless conversations where it has been absolutely vital for me to listen, process, acknowledge and respond adequately but I have been unable to do most of it because I am too distracted by my inner emotions.

Worse still, if I am assailed by many feelings, I don't show it on the outside. If I am feeling overwhelmed, then I am more likely to appear bored or sound monotone. It's a strange paradox that the greater the tumult within, the duller the outside of me often becomes, so that I appear as if I was barely operating at all.

You can imagine the effect this has on the other person in the conversation. They are telling me the essential details of their personal life and I look like they're reading and re-reading the menu from a truck stop.

Do you know, I feel as interested as if they *are* reading that menu. Sad as it is, the emotional wreckage going on within and without means that not only do I look disinterested and idle, I also feel it.

How can I be anything else, though? I have so much pestering me for attention that there is very little of me left over to counsel you on how best to manage Dave and his obnoxious step-son. Perhaps if you come back next week I can offer more advice? Or maybe you should have taken the advice I gave you last time, when I was in a better frame of mind? You could have told Dave exactly what Daniel did with his telescope and why he now has a police record.

Still, the good thing about being overwhelmed by feelings is that these conversations are often cut short and I am free to calm down and remove myself to a safe place, away from the whole stupid, awful, noisy, feeling-full portion of life which I had to endure for the last twenty hours (ten minutes).

Unfortunately, this usually doesn't happen as my non-reaction has been received as non-caring and I am now the enemy, the person who should be helping but is so bored and horrible they can't even get beyond one syllable answers to life's important questions.

The guilt is brought in on a gold platter, pulled by shiny page-boys and presented to me as a prize, another time I have let people down and gone away with even more negative feelings which stop me presenting my good side during conversations.

After the event, when I have looked at it all again and realised I was overwhelmed and should have been more attentive, I may try to put things right and apologise. All too late, of course. The conversation is a finite event, stuck in time; it doesn't wait for me to come back to it or be ready to pay attention. It goes on without me, taken by the winds of regret and lost forever. Anything I say on the matter now will be viewed with suspicion and paranoia, as if I am only pretending to care.

There will be no acceptable explanation for my dull conduct during our conversation and I wouldn't be able to verbalise it all anyway. Here, in words, it comes to me and I can tell you everything, but in the middle of real-life when it matters most to me, I stand and stare out of the window, wishing for the quiet of home and wondering when I will ever be able to care enough to listen.

But you should just know...

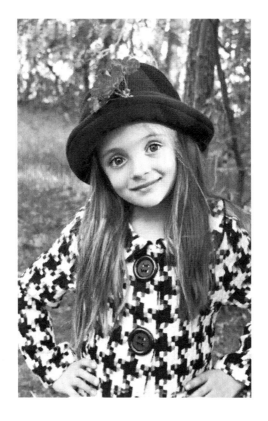

Look, can we get this straight, once and for all? Aspies are not good at taking the hint, especially if the hint is a subtle one. Imagine how hard it is to take a hint that is being hinted, getting all hinty with you, and is then left unspoken because you're meant to be taking the hint! This is what it is like when a non-aspie wants you to know something without actually telling you.

If a person is upset with their aspie, it's so much better to say so and be specific about *why* they are upset. It is no good at all going round like an old piece of flannel, hoping your aspie will notice you're upset or, worse still, realise they are to blame.

If you're very lucky, your aspie will think you look a bit bored, as you haven't been laughing much lately, and perhaps suggest a game of Super Smash Bros Brawl to cheer you up.

At this point, the mood of the non-aspie, hoping for attention, takes a nose-dive as being invited to do something your aspie likes doing is a reminder that your silent upset has gone unnoticed and that the aspie is behaving in their usual selfish way by only wanting to do what they enjoy.

The aspie carries on, quite happy that life is fine and now knowing you can't be too bored or you would have accepted their offer to play a game. They forget all about your glum face and ask you when tea will be ready or immerse themselves in Super Smash Bros Brawl, having decided to play it anyway.

The upset, neglected, hinty non-aspie has two choices at this point. They can either explode, which would be messy or just tell the aspie what is wrong with them. Or, like a big silly child they can take the sulk to the next stage, still waiting for the aspie to know what is wrong. You'll notice there were three choices: really, I'm only giving you two. Do not progress to the next stage of the sulk!

In the world of non-aspies, many things seem to be Known. It's like there is this vast intranet club, connecting all non-aspies, feeding them vast amounts of secret information which they feel is known to everyone. They don't realise they are closed off from the aspie world, connected with a lot of people but not to the aspie sitting next to them.

When something happens and a pattern of behaviour is followed, the non-aspie expects their eccentric, inventive, creative and awkward beloved to know, without being told, what to do next. If the non-aspie is ill, the aspie is expected to be sympathetic and look after them. If they are upset, then the aspie should know they are upset, by their behaviour and little things they say. If the non-aspie is worried about something, their aspie should be able to tell, without them having to be obvious about it.

Sometimes, aspies do know without being told. If you are being sick down the toilet for the third time in one morning, we are not stupid, it is kind of obvious you're not feeling well. It's unlikely we'll want to come and sympathise but we will have noticed.

However, if you are feeling under the weather and a bit icky, don't sit there like Grandpop's sock, expecting us to link to your closed intranet and know you are ill. If we see you sitting there, do you know what we think when your sad, pale little face turns in our direction? We think, Gosh, best beloved doesn't seem to be doing much today, they must be tired. I wonder when tea will be ready?

33

If you are upset and mooch about, clashing pots and pans, slamming doors, generally making it obvious you are upset, do you know what we're thinking? Mostly, we're thinking what a great load of noise you're making when we're trying to concentrate on Facebook or sending an important email or getting past this tricky level in Great Grand and Grizzly on the PlayStation.

If we hear the muttering and start to realise you're being a bit snappy, then we think you've maybe been upset by someone or had a bad day. It doesn't automatically occur to us that *we* are the guilty party because if we were, you'd have said something: wouldn't you?

And if you're worried and hoping we'll notice so you can talk about it? Well, for heaven's sake, just say so! It's no good trooping past with a pained expression. If we do see your face, we'll just think you need the toilet or have a tummy ache and carry on with what we're doing. Again, if you need help, we expect you to ask for it, like we would.

It infuriates me to the jumping-up-and-down stage when other people expect me to Know things. I have come a cropper with this many times and it always ends up being revealed in the middle of some nasty row or silly snapping contest where I'm suddenly told that I *know* what is the matter and am then presented with evidence as to why I know.

The evidence often consists of something forgotten or that happened when I wasn't paying attention. I'm not saying the aspie is innocent in all these matters - often it is our fault, once we get to the bottom of it. But if people would just say what is wrong, instead of relying on silly conventions of behaviour where we are all meant to know the rules for unspoken communication, then life would be a whole lot simpler.

For the record, I do think it's appropriate to cheer someone up by offering to play a video game with them - it always cheers *me* up - so I think grumpy-groos could cut me a little slack and not use the offer of a game against me, along with my other wrongdoings.

Other aspies will have their own examples to fill in here, their own wrongdoings too. It's all relative, all individual, according to the aspie and their friends and family. What seems to remain a constant is the ability of so-called normal people to make the aspie life way more complicated than it ever needs to be.

As I have said before, if you need me to know something, just tell me!

High emotions

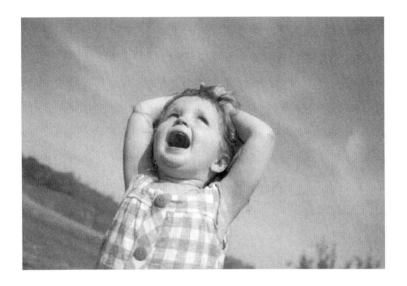

Usually, a state of high emotion seems to hurt like nettle rash or pins and needles, at that stage when your foot is trying to recover and you don't know whether to hop about like a mad thing or sit very still until it stops hurting. It's not something I seek out and given the choice between emotional pins and needles or the calm of neutral feelings, then I know which I would choose.

There is something very soothing about keeping high emotions at bay; it's like you've discovered a secret to the universe as you gaze at other people scurrying to and fro, as if the being-busy is all there is to human life and an end in itself.

I've been accused in the past of being cold and unfeeling. Not so, I feel things very much, though I couldn't always describe to you how I feel or how I want to react. With Aspergers, it often seems to be show rather than tell. If you want to know how I feel about something, pay attention and I'll show you - don't ask me to describe it in words.

I think this comes to mind most when I am bothered about something and don't know why. My emotions then are not calm and I start the helter-skelter of going round and down and having no idea exactly why I react the way I do. Often this sudden downswing and feeling of instability is caused by something minor, totally out of proportion with the reaction I have.

I sometimes ask my friend why I should feel the way I do, knowing she has the objectivity and wisdom to say: *this* is what bothers you about it, *this* is why you are upset. It's very important to have someone who can tell you these things, especially if they know you well.

It's a little like having an interpreter who can explain to you what life means when it mixes with what goes on inside you. Aspies are very good at reactions but not so good at unravelling the reasons behind them. And it can be very important to unravel these reactions if you are creating a situation where your emotional response is about to involve more than yourself or have consequences.

And there is the crux of a great deal of aspie angst: we feel we should be doing something or behaving in a certain way when we're not usually capable of doing so. We are what we are, we will never be other people.

Some don't look at the stars and see the heavens, they see the night and hurry home.

We shouldn't try to be like other people and, by association, we shouldn't expect to act like them. Our feelings of prickly high emotion, so unwelcome in the aspie-verse, are often caused by unrealistic expectations, brought on by us thinking we should be something other than what we are or can be.

As I often say, we should be kind to ourselves, even if it sometimes means letting people down. There is only so much that can be done and too much suffering is brought on by hoping or expecting to suddenly change into a different person who can do all the things we never could before.

High emotions are positive, in the right situation and with goodness in them. What we don't want is the feeling of pain coming with them, of the foot being too hot as it wakes so that we need to rub it, hard and all at once, to make it normal again.

There is enough harshness in the world without inviting it in. Coolness of temper and softness of emotion are more preferable than the feeling that you must suffer to make something right.

Aspies are Fools

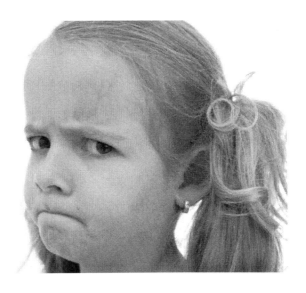

April Fool's Day is an invention designed to make a certain portion of society feel like they should know better than to get out of bed in the morning. Once people pass an age when eating worms is fun, playing April Fool's tricks is more an exercise in wilful cruelty than a light-hearted joke.

This April was no different, with 'funnies' going on all over the internet (and yes, some are funny) and lots of fake statuses on Facebook (no change there then). I was drawn in more by the statuses as it's natural to read them and think they're really what people are thinking and doing.

I expect it seems silly to the less gullible that I wouldn't automatically think of April Fool's when I was reading these things. I did. I reminded myself of the date before I logged on but forgot as soon as I was immersed.

It's very annoying as my first reaction is to believe the status, then the second reaction is to realise they're not being serious. My third reaction is to feel ashamed that I was caught out again, even though no one knows.

I hate that feeling, the creeping shame that I got it wrong on such an obvious, elementary level. It's not because I'm full of pride, I don't mind laughing at myself. It's more to do with all the times when it happens accidentally, when other people say something and I don't realise they're either joking or lying and I get taken in.

Again and again, readers. How many times do you have to be gullible before it wears off? Does it ever? Would I want it to?

I often think of myself as cynical when it comes to some parts of life but when other people open their mouths and say something, I tend to believe them before I think it through. It's as if the words tumbling from their lips form their own kind of reality. It is true because it was spoken.

Then I have to backtrack and remind myself that people often say things that aren't true. I know this is not news but still I expect others to tell the truth. Knowing that people lie and then applying that to the person standing in front of you are two different things.

Yet it happens so often I should be used to it. I don't mean I'm surrounded by liars, or that they are all false friends. Perhaps it's easier to say I often feel surrounded by people who massage reality, to try and get it to do what they want.

Also, they assume everyone else does the same and see nothing wrong with blending truth and lies. If I am taken in, it is my fault.

This is the accepted wisdom. Just as on April Fool's Day, there is a type of Buyer Beware running through life where the liar, the naysayer, the flimsy-worded malcontent who would have you treat them as a friend, thinks that if you believe what they say then it is your fault.

Doesn't everyone bend the truth? Therefore if we believe everything we are told, we must be fools. Somewhere along the line it became a given fact that people who take everyone as they see them and expect honesty are gullible and naive, whereas those who twist their words are people who live in the real world.

This real world of which you speak, it is nothing more and nothing less than real. Words cannot change it and small, imperceptible lies won't change it either.

I am a fool who thinks each new person may be honest, even though I know many people are not. I am still gullible after all these years and can be taken in by soft voices and smiling faces. I am naive and believe that people can be my friend, right here and now, because it feels like friendship.

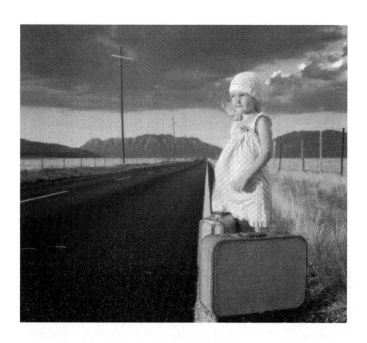

Each day may have a breath of April Fool's to it but it's far better to live this way than to be always struggling in a morass of what is and is not true. Lying, to yourself or the world at large is a lifelong commitment. Being a fool comes naturally and makes every day feel like new.

2: Confusion

Aspies are not always confused but confusion is a constant background feature of living with Aspergers. We do not set out to be confused by life, we actually endeavour to understand life, all the time. Yet still confusion is the primary response when we are faced with something complex.

This is understandable but when you apply being confused with complex issues, it has to be understood that my complex issues and yours may not be the same. A massively emotional situation is complex but so is a visit to the dentist. An argument with half my family is very complex and confusing; so how can I apply the same confusion to one phone call or a conversation with someone who cares?

Life is complex and life is confusing. To someone with Aspergers, tiny parts of life are difficult to tease out and we feel the same confusion as a non-aspie might experience in a much more tangled situation.

It is maddening to have this confusion with us all the time! Imagine how it feels to wonder about normal, everyday scenarios or be bamboozled by the inexplicable actions of our nearest and dearest. And then be told we are being silly, that it is all commonplace, that everyone understands this so how can we not?

This section is about how confusion winds its way into communication, causing more problems and creating that chaos of which we should be fond, seeing as we spend so much time with it.

Forgetfulness

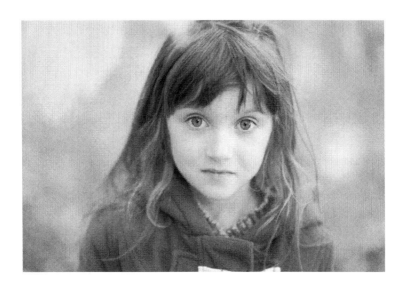

There is something particularly off-putting about being asked a question to which you know the answer. It's happened to us all, you feel you knew something right up until the moment you were asked to share it. The name of an actor, the book you read last week, that girl you went to school with who ended up living with three men. You know, all the stuff your brain stored away for when it would be useful.

At first I thought I was reacting to stress, especially as this forgetfulness seemed to happen more over the last couple of years when normal life hasn't been that easy. Then I thought I was probably tired - so much can be blamed on this that it almost starts to feel like a vendetta to blame Tired again. Oh, it's Tired's fault, Tired made me do it, I'm just feeling Tired.

47

Then I decided I was actually suffering from distraction, as a separate concept. Yes, I did. even though I've arguably suffered from distraction my whole life (I believe they call it not fulfilling your potential). I decided that distraction was to blame for the new heights of forgetfulness. I was distracted by (insert anything) and then I forgot. Or, my brain is working on so many levels at the same time, I forgot this part.

Yes, sounds like an excuse. It begins to feel like forgetting is a way of expressing other problems in life. Tired leads to it, Distraction, Stress, whatever is bothering you at the time. When do I stop and take a closer look? When does it become a problem by itself?

Well, when you also forget on those days where everything is going right and you've had enough sleep and are completely relaxed and there is no earthly reason why you should forget what you needed to remember. That's when forgetfulness finally claims your attention in its own right.

Like the little quiet child at the back of the class, forgetfulness has been raising her hand every time you wanted to know the answer and you kept going for silly Distraction and over-achieving Stress and even choosing gloomy Tired. When were you ever going to see pretty little Forgetfulness, dressed in blue with flowers in her hair? Hasn't she been trying to help you all this time by giving you the answer?

Yes, readers, she has been trying to help me because I've come to the conclusion Forgetfulness and I should be friends and see what we can do for each other.

When I am sitting in my lessons, waiting to help a student and I forget what I have known for twenty five years then I no longer blame Distraction and co. I see it for what it is, Forgetfulness stretching her legs and enjoying the sun. What she wanted to do today was play, you see, and so even though you had enough sleep and no distractions and were feeling relaxed, you still forgot what you needed to know because Forgetfulness thought this was a fine day to lounge in the imagination and not be present in real life.

Striding through town, intent on your errands, you might blame the others for taking you right past the stationery shop again. When will you ever remember the printer paper? Will you have to start printing on toilet paper before you buy some? No, it was Forgetfulness, enjoying the striding through town, enjoying the feeling of walking with purpose and having somewhere to go. Forgetfulness only remembered going to the chemist because that meant more striding; she wasn't really interested in the little jobs like essential paper.

So, how does Forgetfulness help? It really sounds as if she is a gentle but troublesome child who wants to do only what interests her at the time and forgets the rest. Well, there you have it.

If you remember everything you have to do, Stress creeps in. If you have too much to do and lots going on in your life, Distraction jumps out from behind a door to surprise you then invites you to a game of chess to take your mind off things. If you are dragging yourself through too much today and then don't sleep because you had to cope with more than was healthy,

Tired gets up with you in the morning and leans on your arm all day, slowing you down because Tired just can't be bothered.

Forgetfulness to the rescue! She knows those other students all claim too much of your attention. She knows she is quiet and that you don't always listen to her but she also knows where the stream plays through the wood and the light falls between the trees. She knows where you can lie and watch the world pass by. No one will ever see where Forgetfulness takes you.

She knows you must be rested, right here and now, even when you think you have rested enough. She takes your hand and leads you a little distance away from what you were doing then lets you go back, a small amount of her peace going with you.

Forgetfulness remembers less than you would like and she does it on purpose. We don't always need those big meltdowns or unequivocal slamming of doors to shut out the outside world. We don't always want to spend days conquering a new computer game as a way of avoiding real-life problems. We don't always want to pile up our to-do list until it is a teetering, unmanageable slope.

What we need is to learn to leave, presently and momentarily, in the middle of what we are doing. Pause, readers, and refresh. Come back, apologise for your absence then try again.

On the best and strongest of days there is nothing wrong with forgetting, even for a few seconds. It is our way of reminding ourselves, of remembering we are dancing through this life with one step always in mid-air, wondering where it will come down. We cannot dance if we are tired, stressed and distracted.

Forgetfulness helps us ignore all of them and dance anyway.

Aspie imagination vs real life

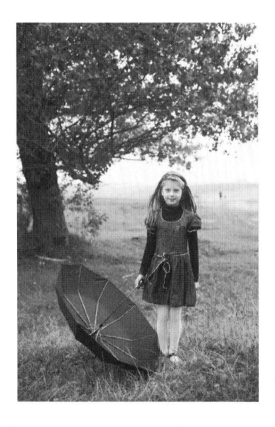

It's all very well me going on about how much imagination we aspies have, when I know that being able to visualise things is far from the same thing as being able to understand them. Sometimes this visualisation can cause more problems than it solves. After all, visualising being eaten by a giant bear does nothing to help you cross the forest. If anything, it's more likely to make you stay indoors and never cross the forest again.

In a similar way, aspies often find themselves imagining the bad things that can happen. These bad things may start off small but like nasty little acorns they grow and grow until all you see is the very thing you wanted to avoid in the first place. This obsessive quality of the aspie links very neatly with the ability to imagine the worst and create something all-consuming.

Social situations would be a really good example of this. The fear is already there so it doesn't take much of a nudge from my imagination for me to start seeing how it could all go wrong, with me at the centre of the wrongness. Sometimes, when the event (or torture) is over, I can look back and know that it was all imagination, that it turned out pretty well in the end. But mostly, how it turns out means very little because even though your imagined prediction didn't come true, you know it might the next time and, logically, if not then, *one* of those times will be as horrible as you imagined.

Yes, it is ridiculous in a way, to make ourselves suffer like this and we are creating an impossible problem. If the dreaded scenarios we come up with don't happen, we are still convinced they can and might the next time. Taking that as a rule for preparing for social interactions means we will always have the fear of what can go wrong and never be free of it.

If we follow this rule, it won't matter how often it goes right or for how long: we will still, no matter what, be waiting for it to go wrong and then, if it does, we'll know we were right to worry.

You see, alongside any dramatic and creative difficulties we make for ourselves, the fear is always there so it often *feels* as though it went wrong, even if it didn't. We can't relax and form enough confidence to carry us through to the next time.

If you can approach social situations without this worry, then you are free to enjoy them and it probably won't occur to you to worry each time you have to interact with people. Imagine if the opposite was true, though: that each situation is stressful, despite any enjoyment you have and each future interaction has the potential to worry you for days before it happens.

It's one of the more frustrating aspects of Aspergers that past experience only goes so far in smoothing down the corners of harsh and unforgiving worry. It's very easy for aspies to use past stresses and unhappy situations to prove to themselves that the next will be just as bad but it's very difficult to use past *happy* outcomes as reassurance that it will be good next time too.

It doesn't necessarily have anything to do with how often things go right or wrong, either. It has more foundation in our self-image, as we expect to get things wrong and if you don't have confidence in yourself, then why should you have any in other people or the world around you?

I'm painting aspies as a gloomy bunch, like Eeyore, waiting for the worst to happen and knowing it will, if you wait long enough. It isn't like that, honestly. We are full of many emotions and reactions besides the dread and real life does go on around us while we're imagining the worst.

Simply put, we are conscious of how transient the steady, stable feelings can be because life is so confusing at times, and surprising too. We know how very quickly we find things tipped on their heads with us wondering where our feet are meant to be.

You see, it doesn't take much for us to believe we've got it wrong again or that the expected problems occurred. I've used social interactions as an example because they cause me so many difficulties but they are a problem for many aspies because they bring us into contact with other people.

When it comes to our imaginations creating scary potential scenarios, it doesn't come much scarier than imagining what other people might do. Even for the sociable aspie, people are the most confusing element in life. They behave erratically, unpredictably and sometimes cruelly. They say things we don't expect and behave in ways that make no sense.

People are easy to offend and upset, even when we try our best. They come out with statements that seem to bear no relation to what is happening and then expect us to know what it's all about. The most friendly of people can still cause problems simply by approaching us as if we know all the same things they do.

Aspies are often on their guard, ready for people to throw a curve ball, as if they're playing a friendly game of catch in the park. How are we meant to catch the ball when we didn't even know you had it in your hand until it was hurtling through the air?

We have to keep our reactions and attentions focussed on other people to make sure there are no unwanted surprises. This is why we often appear odd or disconnected. We spend so much time reacting, processing and keeping our attention on the here and now.

Frankly, having Aspergers can often feel like being a few people at once, as if you were more than one version of yourself, existing in the same space and time but ever so slightly out of sync so that if you move too fast or the world tilts, everything blurs and you lose coherence for a moment.

You try negotiating normal, everyday life, with all that going on inside you. It makes life interesting, to say the least. If I seem distracted and surprised at any time, consider the fact that it can be quite hard to keep a grip on what you are doing and saying and expecting of me, when I can barely hold on to what I expect of myself.

In the end, I don't want you to leave thinking that I and other aspies are a bunch of stressed-out miseries, who can't string a sentence together because we're too busy dealing with sensory overload. You know, we're quite used to the way we are, we often only run into problems when the world around us behaves unexpectedly.

All you need to do is give us a little catch-up time and not be flinging that ball through the air, wondering why it bounces right off our forehead and disappears into the bushes. Games of catch, like life itself, are best played when everyone is in the same place and aware of the same things. Give us a little warning and we may try to catch the ball. Or we may not. Catch always seemed like a pointless game to me, so why not put the ball away and come and play a different game?

Communication is like a bucking bronco

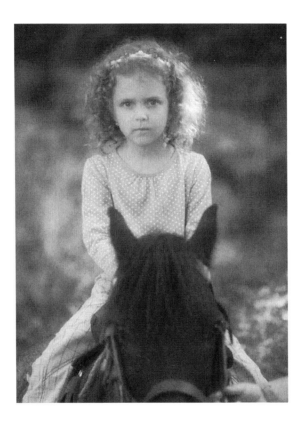

There are two things needed for an honest conversation and only one of them is honesty itself.

The second thing you need, a vital ingredient to making the honesty work, is the ability to express yourself. Without this ability, honesty becomes just a momentary bolt for the door, or a brief splurge of feelings, as and when they happen.

It's rather like saying to the bread dough, 'Now, Dough, I've held up my part of the bargain: you have yeast, an oiled bowl and I've kneaded you straight through five songs and an ad break on the radio. Whenever the heck are you going to start rising?'

The bread would feel even more deflated at this, having no idea why it can't rise. Imagine the sad lump of dough in the bowl, still not touching the sides, still as you left it an hour ago. What can it be doing wrong?

The bread knows you did everything you could. It knows about the yeast, the bowl, the kneading. It remembers the endless radio noise as you went to work. It realises that now all it has to do is hold up one small part of the bargain and rise.

What it doesn't know and what you forgot is that it needs some warmth too.

Without warmth, you will probably get some rising, eventually. It wasn't the dough's fault that you forgot it needed warmth, it only understands part of the process.

Okay, aspies are not bread dough, though we also require some warmth to grow. What I am trying to explain is, we rarely have the full picture, not when it comes to ourselves.

Sometimes, we desperately want to express ourselves and be honest and all we manage is a small sentence on how we aren't feeling too good. Often we divert and think we are ill instead, thanks to the twisting stomach and the frantic headache brought on by nerves.

Someone else might need to step in and remind us why we don't feel happy or to ask pointed, direct questions to get to the heart of the matter. It is no good expecting answers when you haven't asked the right questions. How many times have I wondered, long after the event, what someone really wanted to know after a conversation with them! If only they had come out and said, without expecting me to remember or *know*.

If you would like to know how an aspie feels, ask and risk rejection or horror or the sight of heels disappearing in the opposite direction. But also be prepared to prompt and help along the conversation.

Do not push in and say, 'But you said you were desperate to go to Valencia!' only to have your aspie remember, quite clearly, that it was *you* who was desperate for a holiday in the sun. Try instead, 'What exactly worries you about Valencia?' (I have nothing against Valencia, by the way, feel free to go on holiday there with my blessing).

Be brave and ask questions, be forthright - give honesty in the hopes of receiving it. And do not, in any way, play games, expecting your aspie to know what their part is or that anyone is playing at all in the first place.

Above all, remember that communication is a constantly evolving, tumultuous beast, only dressed blithely in summer clothes because the human race decided communication had to be a civilised thing. In real, human relationships, where people want to communicate, not just get along or pretend to be friends, then communication is a primeval and vital component, ever-changing to suit the needs of the moment. It must be ridden like the bronco, steered as well as you can, holding on and feeling for the next move before it even happens.

This, after all, is what communication is like for aspies most days of the week. Try it in its basic, pre-dawn form and see how well you get on. At the very least, you'll start to see each other in a new light. Being kicked off into the dirt can do that for you.

Aspies, masters of the awkward question

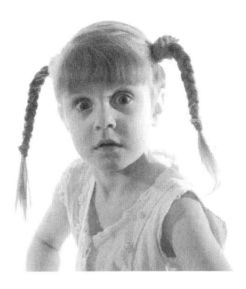

I don't usually mean to be rude or even impolite. I try to be pleasant and respectful, even in the face of extreme provocation. If pushed, I'm more likely to resort to unexpected sarcasm or pointing out (helpfully) how and why you went wrong. I'm rarely out-and-out bad mannered.

So, it often comes as a surprise when people react as if I spat on their foot. I mean it, this is as close an analogy as I can think of to describe the sudden backwards flinch, with the lip rising in thinly-veiled horror. I do want to be clear - I haven't spat on their foot, and if I tried, I would definitely miss.

What I have done is Enter into a Conversation. I do often warn myself off this as it ends badly or chugs along nicely until I replay it afterwards and realise I had it all wrong and gave a strange impression (again). In trying to speak to someone in a normal way, I'll do what comes naturally: ask questions.

I'm interested, you see. If someone has my attention, they are already winning and if they are managing to keep my attention, the conversation can't be half bad. So it is only natural for me to want to learn more and ask pertinent questions. This is a compliment!

What I don't always understand is that the other person only wants to talk and not really interact. They want to tell me their news or carry on with their diatribe without me butting in and stopping the narrative flow by being a part of the conversation.

Although I'll be asking a question that is wholly relevant, they still see it as a burden to have to slow down and answer it before continuing. Or they wave it away and promise to come back to it (but never do).

I've thought about this and realise the other person isn't interested in me fully understanding their subject of conversation - they only want superficial understanding so that they can rattle on without me piping up in the middle of it. This means that me asking a question which requires an answer - rather than a rhetorical one, which helps the flow - is an awkward bump on the road which means they have to divert or slow down.

Their other issue is that if they do have my full attention, I won't be put off when I ask the question. I *must* know the answer! If I didn't want to know the answer then I probably wouldn't have asked. And if they don't reply, or fudge the answer hoping to throw me off track, I'll come back, quick as lickety-split and ask again, assuming they haven't understood what I want to know.

You see, if I have a full conversation with someone about a subject I'm interested in and know about, I love it if the other person asks a question. It shows they share my enthusiasm or want to know more. And I rarely get diverted for long from my subject so answering a question becomes part of the rich landscape of that whole conversation.

I'm not sure how I'm meant to tell the difference between someone who wants to have a proper conversation, or someone who just wants to hear the sound of their own voice and use me as a convenient audience at the time. How do you know before putting your foot in it and asking questions they don't want to answer?

Also, the consequence of them behaving in this way is that if they don't answer my question, or they try to power on as if I haven't spoken, then I'm very likely to leave the conversation altogether, either by developing a sudden (and inventive) excuse or just walking off.

Readers, it's not my fault if people can't cope when their audience departs to the bar, or out the back door or starts to pick up the first soft tomato. People should be more aware of what they are getting into when they invite an aspie to talk to them. Don't they know how risky it can be to perform to such a brutally honest and direct audience?

Well, if they don't at the start of the show, they certainly do by the end.

Snap! Putting names to faces

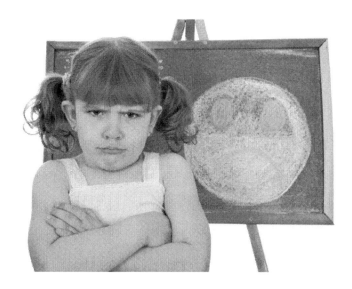

Someone walks towards you, a half-smile on their lips. You run the smile through various internal algorithms and find it could be that they know you, they want to know you or they have an axe behind their back.

Erring on the side of caution, you smile back, uncertainly. They stop and begin to talk. It's obvious they know you. Searching their face for clues, you come up with

aspie-recog-failure error code nn231

In other words, you don't recognise them, either at all or enough to remember how you're supposed to react.

From the way they're talking to you, they seem to know quite a bit about you and your personality. This is a relief as it means you can talk back and generally be yourself without worrying too much about putting your foot in it.

All the while, you're looking at them, assessing what they say, working though the variables. What they say, does it match with a potential friend of a friend or a past colleague or boss? (No, you always remember the bosses, unfortunately). Was it someone who knew you in school and who has changed enough for you not to know them?

Worrying thoughts cascade. In my experience, as quite an anti-social aspie, I've still come across many people because of all the jobs I've done, so when someone seems to know me I always re-visit past colleagues first.

Eventually, they move on, happy to have caught up with you. Watching them go, you're happy that you didn't walk past them and maybe hurt their feelings or leave another person wondering at how strange you are.

This is all part of the great dance of recognition which many aspies have trouble with. It's not just about remembering, or forgetting, people you once knew. We can all do that. It's about not knowing the ones who should still be familiar.

In the past, I've had a friend jump up and down in the street when she saw me coming, having exhausted all other ways of getting my attention besides hitting me over the head with something. She even shouted my name. Not a thing had registered. The jumping up and down *did* register and we laughed about it. She wasn't worried, she knew I wouldn't ignore her on purpose and was happy to do whatever it took to speak to me.

I know I've ignored others over the years. I'm attuned to the odd, sideways glance you get from people who think you're ignoring them. Attuned to *that* but not to recognising them in the first place!

It comes down to people you're close to or who have known you well. Readers, I'm embarrassed to admit it but I once followed a strange man down two streets before I worked out it wasn't my ex-husband. I did wonder why he kept hurrying off.

I've heard it called facial blindness but I prefer to think of it as a recognition problem because it extends well beyond the face. It's down to how you *expect* a person to look, given what they looked like before.

If they appear in front of you, wearing the same things and sporting the same hairstyle as when you last saw them, then you're very, very much more likely to know them. They're programmed in as Nigel, curly-hair, two children, likes trains.

If you come across Nigel six months later and he's had a close shave, he might be familiar still or he might have to come right up and start talking about trains for you to know who it is.

A clue might lie in how we perceive the world, with our over-load of information. As we're always trying to weigh things up and work them out, the physical appearance of a person is also filed under available information. We use it to match them up in our minds.

The problem lies in the fact that if we were to meet them walking down the street inside our heads, we would know them instantly, as we have their features on file and it's all close to hand. Out in the world, with so many other distractions to cope with, a person has to fight with life itself to gain your attention and have you know them. A taller order.

Here's another one: I do think that we see people as snapshots in our internal film reel. There they go, there's Nigel speeding into the distance, hair bobbing in the wind, immortalised forever as he once was. How many times will he feature in the film reel as a different person, later recognised? Does he become a different person each time we meet him? Is he processed as a new encounter until recognised as otherwise?

Just to confuse matters and make myself sound even more complicated, let's look at twins. I'm sorry, there is no such thing as an identical twin to me. Yes, I may pass a best friend in the street and not see her but I can always tell the difference between twins.

At first meeting, I have to really check to see if they are identical. Half the time it doesn't occur to me that they are. IT Teen showed me a video of Dan is not on fire (search YouTube without small children in the room). Dan made a video with his two friends. I worked out after a minute that they were probably brothers, as they looked quite alike - it's hard to tell when they're wearing different clothes. Eventually, yes, you guessed it, I realised they were twins. Or *probably* twins. I checked with IT Teen, who was irritated that I'd obviously been working out the twinship in the video instead of actually watching it.

IT Teen also knows twins who went to the same infant school as him. They do like to dress almost the same, with different colours. To me, it's obvious who is who, they're very distinct people. To IT Teen and the rest of his cohorts, the twins are identical. Sigh.

So, at least the twins of the world can breathe easy that I'm not one of those people who will look from one to the other and say, 'Barry? or is it Buddy?', at least not after the first meeting. No, I'll be the strange lady asking them if they're related.

So, what to do about normal non-recognition? Nothing, actually. I've tried for years to make it work for me and now I've given in to it. If I'm in a crowded place, I'm likely to not recognise people. If I do, I may not know from where. If they recognise me first, I will speak and talk and have a conversation to the best of my abilities.

I'm not yet brave enough to smile sweetly and ask who they are. Too much risk of hurt feelings - it's not their fault I don't know them. It's not mine, either, as it's a side-effect of being an aspie. But all this would take too long to explain and their feelings would already be hurt by then so I just leave it.

The only advice I can give is, if really pushed, 'fess up and say, 'I'm sorry, my memory is terrible, what was your name again?'

If you can do it with ease, making it all about *yourself* and not them, the feelings are usually avoided. Personally, I'm rubbish at this kind of thing and would give them a sickly smile while I did it, making it obvious I suspect them of being an imposter who I have never, in my life, met before.

The most I can say is, this recognition error in the aspie psyche is one area that no amount of effort or self-chastisement will fix. So, there should be no guilt with it either. This one, we have to accept. Just do your best not to offend people and use it as practice for talking to anyone who talks to you. Sometimes you won't know them and they'll just be the friendly type but it never hurts to make new friends.

Of course, the next time you see them you'll have no idea where you met them before. Was it the job at the zoo? Are they friends with Stella? You never liked Stella. Didn't she have strange taste in men...Oh! They're still talking! Now, where do I know them from???

Seeing things through aspie eyes

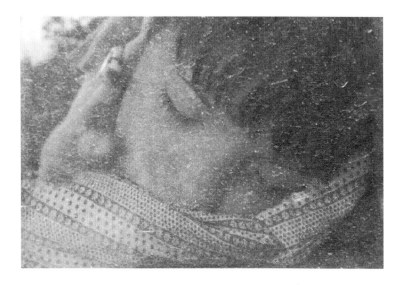

Imagine a toy box full of bricks. They're the building bricks kind with those little house shapes so you can make your very own town. All brightly coloured and smart, brand new from the shop. How lovely they look, inviting and begging small hands to take them out and play!

Then the box is tipped over, sending bricks, houses, tiny wooden cars and all the shapes you love are sent tumbling across the floor. They scatter, some landing in heaps, others rolling off next to the door. They are everywhere and this is how toddlers like them: all over the place, ready to be picked up one-by-one as needed.

These bricks don't belong in the box, you see, where they look neat and gleaming in the light from the nursery window; they belong on the floor so little hands can choose them without having to rummage through a massive pile to find what they need.

You have a happy, unconcerned toddler on the floor, choosing bricks and building their own little world. And then the aspie toddler arrives.

Mess everywhere! Colours streaming in the air as if the bricks were in constant motion, their tumble from the box continuing in the aspie mind as the colours and shapes jumble together and become a mass of confusion.

It doesn't matter that each brick is now separate and easier to choose: all at once, there are too many. They are only easier to choose for the non-aspie toddler who can look at them and see only fun.

To the aspie toddler they are now too many, their pieces noisy and crowded, the room full of disturbance like the air when it is full and heavy before a storm. The bricks, shining in the sunlight, seem to sneer and crackle at the aspie, daring a touch, raging at the quiet air, too loud and bright for a safe encounter.

If the bricks are in their box, the aspie toddler knows where to find them. He knows if he digs deep, he will be able to push past the bricks he doesn't need to find the one he does. Taking the trouble to search is nothing compared to the shock of having them all laid out at once, challenging him to put aside the distraction of so many pieces. Far better to dig and know what you are looking for than to be presented with the whole of choice and forget what you needed to find.

The aspie toddler sets to and starts to gather the bricks. At first the non-aspie ignores him, thinking his friend is joining in the game. Once he sees that aspie means to put away all the bricks there is sorrow and anger. They're supposed to be out there like that! It's part of the game!

Aspie ignores the noises from his friend, barely registers anything except the need to replace the bricks. Once the bricks are away and all in their right place, then it will be good again. The sunlight will be just bright enough and the nursery floor will look how it is meant to, without the clutter of too many distractions.

There is a tussle as non-aspie tries to stop the aspie replacing the bricks. Finally aspie realises that non-aspie doesn't want them away and, worse still, will most likely tip them out again as soon as they are tidy. A quick, sharp flash of fear fills the aspie toddler as he sees his work is in vain: the bricks will come back out and be disassembled, all his work undone and confusion permanent.

He steps away, face creasing in sadness and the beginnings of panic. He wails as he steps on one of the loose bricks and looks at non-aspie's uncomprehending face. It will never be safe in the nursery, he will never be able to keep all the bricks in their rightful place. He will always be at the door, unable to work out where to step safely or which brick to pick up first.

Tears streaming, he runs for the door, stumbling on his way over the bricks and reaching for the safety of the hall outside. Falling through, the light of the nursery is left behind, dwindled to a glimmering crack in the door. Through the gap he can hear non-aspie taking out the bricks he put away and playing happily. His heart dreads returning and yet longs to be in there, wanting to understand why the mess is safe and not wonder what comes next.

He turns his face to the door, plucking up the courage to go in and try again. This time, he will succeed.

3: It's more than talking

There is so much more to communication than talking (unfortunately!). Getting the hang of the spoken word is difficult enough; trying to grasp all the extra nuances of tone, body language, circumstance, personal ambition and of the ways that communication is altered by context can be impossible.

Talking is awkward as people often don't say what they mean. Try adding in that they have a head ache, that they spilled milk on their way out of the house, that the last time you saw them you insulted their mother and then complete the scenario by being distracted by a droning noise from somewhere to the West and you have a recipe for disaster.

You can complicate it further by having a difficult history with the person or you have disengaged your brain from your mouth that day. Anything and everything can affect even the most well-intentioned aspie to the point where we dread conversations and communication becomes a minefield.

This section draws in those other elements of communication, the aspects of life which make talking almost secondary to real dialogue. Aspies have great problems with setting words in context so extra dimensions of communication can seem unintelligible. And yet, bring your communication back to being 'just' words, such as online messaging or texts and we can rediscover the type of social happiness non-aspies have kept to themselves for years.

We're living in the Age of the Aspie

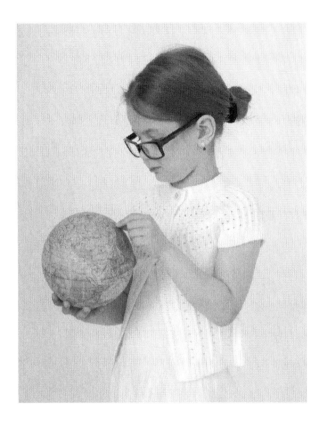

Forget about naming the modern age after anything we've invented, blown up or claimed for our own: until we colonise Mars, the most defining thing about our modern age is the nature of humanity's relationships within itself. And that is why I'm renaming our times as The Age of the Aspie.

In days gone by, in the Western World, stiff manners seemed to be everything. No matter what you did behind closed doors, you had to greet people in the right way and present yourself as an upstanding member of society.

It was all about being seen to do the right thing. You had to be polite, hold down a steady job (or look after the home). Everyone knew their place and that place was unlikely to change, even if you made more money or became a success in other ways.

Even when you moved into the more modern, outwardly permissive, undoubtedly socially-mobile era, there were still expectations of how people would behave. Society as a whole had guidelines and it was your choice if you lived within or without them.

As time shifted towards our present day, computers flourished and seemed to become part of everyone's life, whether they wanted them or not. Here, just *here*, with the mouse connected to the computer, came the emergence of the aspie as a force in everyday life.

I don't mean the mass release of computer geeks all over the world, a naturalisation process hampered only by the uneven divide between the sexes. I don't even mean the way the internet took over everything, suddenly, while no one was looking, aided and abetted by aspies everywhere.

While many aspies have found their calling in the world of computers and technology, I want to point to a lesser-noticed but very important change in society at large.

Once you have a look at the way things have changed, the manners, the expectations, basically everything that makes up society and communication in the modern world, I think it is now an **aspie** world.

It doesn't matter if you are on the spectrum, your communications are likely to be mechanical at times, disjointed, governed by the expectation that all information shared will be in a format suitable for email, Facebook, Twitter or video blog.

If you used to call Aunty Mabel to ask about her bad arm, you're now likely to text her instead and hope the old dear can use her other arm to text you back. Heaven forsake the unlucky friend or relative who is unwilling to embrace this new technology: they'll find themselves wondering why the phone is so quiet these days, even while they receive those annoying beeps on the mobile Betty or Joe got them for Christmas.

Anyone who shuns the modern world and doesn't imbibe of Facebook, email or (I hesitate to type it) *doesn't go online*, will find they still end up talking about these things with the vast majority of people. They'll try to talk about what they read in the newspaper and be given the kind of look reserved for a Penny Farthing rolling down the street. Or there might be a confused moment where the other person asks, 'You mean the Times online?'

The modern world is all about instant information, instant reaction, everyone talking about the same things at the same time or lots of different things with the same people. It is an aspie paradise, full of information to be shared with other enthusiasts and it doesn't ever matter how much you know, there will be a website where you can find out more.

In real life, face to face, aspies will always have their troubles but thanks to the instantaneous nature of the modern world, non-aspies will no longer think it strange if their aspie talks about internet download speed or mentions the latest videos on Reddit. Aspies can talk about these things, more or less safe in the knowledge that the recipient of the conversation will have at least heard of them and probably won't think it's an odd thing to know about.

Conversations themselves are truncated in the modern world, as we rush off to our destinations, mobile phone in hand. People we see on the street, who speak when we meet, are as likely to be Facebook friends as ones we actually know. In fact, it's a relief to see a Facebook friend because having seen their face on screen so many times, we are left in no doubt about who they are and how we relate to them.

Emotions, so rarely displayed in public in the past and such a bugbear for aspies in real life, are now paraded with a whole carnival of dancing butterflies down the main street of online communication. If an aspie is in doubt about how someone is feeling, they can check up on their status, see which pictures they have shared or send them a fun quiz and find out that way.

What was once hidden within is now there for all to see and, best of all, *written down* so that aspies can read it and know what people mean. How strange that if you meet someone in real life and ask how they are, they tell you they're fine but expect you to know if they're not. Online, they tell you everything, whether you want to know it or not and we lucky aspies are not left guessing or trying to work out if we've given the wrong reaction.

And one of the best things of all, readers, is the **delay**. In real life, if someone speaks to you and asks you a question or wants a reaction, it all has to happen *now*. In this one important regard the modern world has slowed things down. When people talk to you online, there is a delay, either while you write back to them or while you pretend to not be online before formulating a response.

So many times I've been caught out by the need for an instant reaction or simply by the look on my face. Online communications, with their in-built delay, are the best advancement in communication our world has ever seen. How many arguments are avoided by people having time to think of the right thing to say instead of the truth?

Yes, I know there are many drawbacks to this modern world of techno-communication. But I tell you, hand on heart, the vast majority of those drawbacks belong to non-aspies. In the aspie world, as well as mostly loving technology, we also love the aspie-spin that has been blended into communication and life in general.

Now, if I get confused, I can Google for the answers. If someone insults me, I can pause before letting fly. If I get a strange email, I can forward it to three different people and have it explained to me. I can look people up, find out what they mean, see what they're feeling today and know them as deeply as is comfortable for me.

And the best thing, yes, the very best thing? Meeting all the other people online who feel the same way and who are willing to consider what we have, with the internet spread out between us, as a proper friendship. The aspie has never been so lucky or so popular as in this modern world, where every day people complain about being displaced and alone.

Readers, until now, it is the aspies who have been displaced and alone. Thanks to the unmanageable speed of modern life, we can now slow down and enjoy the ride. This is what it means to belong.

The unreliable aspie

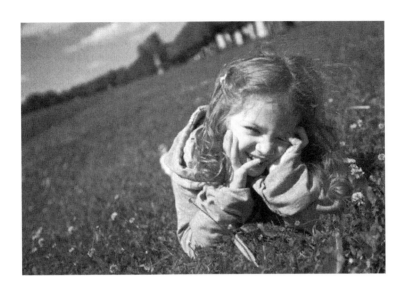

You'd better not ask me to do anything, I'll let you down!

Well, we don't often put it that way, do we? No. Instead we wriggle, and struggle and slip away if possible. Or we have an amazing/totally lame excuse for not doing it - most likely accompanied by the light-bulb expression of just having thought of the excuse.

Okay, so perhaps I'm misjudging you aspies out there? Maybe you're always reliable and can get the job done? Or maybe you *intend* to be reliable and absolutely *know* you can do it? Then, just possibly, something comes up or you have an off day or forget and it still doesn't get done.

So, apologies up-front to any aspies who are reliable and can follow through on their promises. Now, for the rest of us...

How many times have you wanted to help someone and known what you can do to help them, then not done it? This includes either avoiding helping them or saying you will and then not. For me, I wouldn't know anymore. Time and time again, in every area of life.

I'm not proud of it, it's one of the major flaws I see in myself - compared to some of the major flaws I can't see! I mean to do it, have every intention of doing it and then flake out.

It's part of the self-sabotage effect, I think. You don't want to fail so you avoid the issue. Or the thought of being the important part of something is just too unnerving and you back out. Better to let someone else do it than get in the middle, where everyone can see you as you get it wrong.

The agreement to help, the part of you that really does want to come forward and make things better for people, that is genuine. And they will want to accept your help because they'll see the offer is sincere. Your face tells them that, your tone of voice shows them you're there when they need you.

Then when you back out, either a little while before if you're being honest with yourself and know you can't do it or right at the last second if you're still trying to kid yourself; then they see that you aren't reliable and can't be trusted to come through for them. Mistrust sets in and no matter how much they like you or care about you, they don't expect you to be there in times of need.

From this, the seeds of doubt are set in over whether you really care too. If you cared, then you'd be reliable and do what you could to help. This takes a little time to build up, a few failed attempts to gain help from you, a few reasons or excuses given by you that could be true but always seem to come just before you're needed to do something.

It's not surprising if people begin to think you don't care - actions speaking louder than words and all that. If you cared, you'd be there.

This is made worse by what often happens over time: rather than step forward to help, the adult aspie has learned that they're unreliable and becomes less likely to offer help in the first place. This is where the avoidance comes in, leaving the one who needs the help feeling abandoned. Whatever we aspies do, we still come across as not being there when needed.

It doesn't matter how subtle you think you were being either, it's obvious. Don't forget, you're usually dealing with people who can read body language. They don't just listen to what your voice is saying or what you think your face is doing - they see the whole you and they know you're avoiding the issue.

Oh, readers, how often I've stood there at that pivotal point in the conversation, my brain running the conveyor belt at top speed, all the options shooting past of how I could do this and that and then I'd be helping someone. All these things rocket past and I watch them go, knowing if I say anything that we'll all regret it.

I slide off, hoping I got away with it and that no one saw me processing the fact that I could be useful but deciding against it. They don't know I'm avoiding it for their own good. They don't understand that it's better to have this moment of seeming uncaring and selfish than to have the hope bubble float along until I burst it, letting them down far more significantly later.

Am I kidding myself? Do I really just want to be left alone and not help anyone at all? Am I this selfish woman who cares about you only if you don't need anything from me? Sometimes, yes, I think I am that person. The one who lives in her own world and doesn't mind turning her back on the 'real' one.

Mostly, though, these thoughts are sent by me, to punish myself for not being the complete person I imagined I'd be. You're not reliable and you decide you're selfish. You buckle under pressure and call yourself weak. You back out at the last second, unable to face it all, so you must be a horrible person.

One decision leads to another, so one thought process also finds another. This doesn't mean it's all *true*, though. It means, as always, that you're searching for an answer, an explanation that makes sense so that you can look at it, file it away and know it the next time.

It's at odds with the concept of wanting to do something and then doing it. With aspies there is a small crack, just where you step. You intended to go straight from wanting to doing, then flap! your arms are in the air and you're trying to save yourself from falling again.

What to do? Shall I suggest that you be honest and say to someone, 'I don't think I can do that. I'd like to help you, but I don't think I'm able.' This leaves it open, as if you want them to think of a reason why you can do it after all. It sounds like a request.

What about the blunt, honest approach? 'I'm sorry, I can't help you.' Or even just, 'No, I can't help.' Feelings, anyone? They'd be lying on the carpet, gasping for breath by the time you'd finished. But hurt feelings aside, everyone would know exactly where you stood.

Is it better to be brutally honest and get it out of the way than to go along, hoping you can come through this time, only for it to slip out of your grasp again?

On this one, I'm the wrong person to ask. If you'd be able to cope with the reaction you get from complete honesty then go for it but perhaps soften it a little around the edges. If you like, explain somewhat that you find it difficult to help and are tired of letting people down.

I have to admit, if you're like me, you'd still prefer sliding out of the situation, hoping to avoid unnecessary feelings. Let's just leave those feelings alone, shall we? Let's sneak off and pretend we don't know what's happening. Or let's agree and then deal with the consequences later.

Hmm, the more I think about it, the more I see how much simpler it is to be a feelings-thrashing aspie. Honesty first and comfort later. And yet, I'm still not able to do that. Perhaps, when I can be totally honest with myself and admit that I can't face being the one people depend on, then maybe I can start being as honest with those people.

Until then, I'll do what I can, continuing in the hope of being able to help when I say I will because sometimes I do manage it. And then, readers, what a relief to have it out of the way!

Mostly, though, I stand there, face a-twitching, distracted by the noise from that conveyor belt, wondering if I should reach out and pluck something off it or move gently sideways while no one is looking.

When does x become g? and what happened to y?

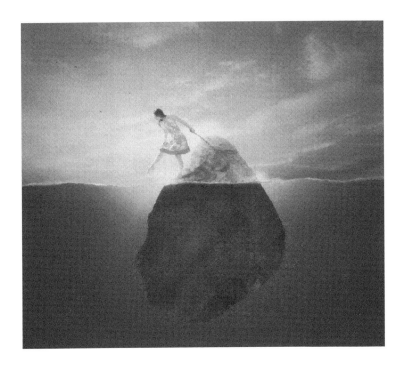

With Aspergers, your own personality and motivations can be as much a mystery as those of other people. With each year that passes, I feel I gain more understanding of myself and I try to make that count in everyday life.

This doesn't always work. A good example would be an argument I had with someone the week before. I can distinctly remember everything that was said and I'm confident I haven't added anything or imagined parts of it as it's so recent. What I find impossible to decipher is why I had the argument in the first place.

It may take the full week, or it may only take sharing it with someone who knows me well, to figure out the secret. Going over the 'facts' such as the conversation itself, reveals some of the puzzle; the rest is either non-verbal, historical problems with the person or even something entirely outside my knowledge.

I've found myself doing this. I look at the words: all okay. I look at the way we've been with each other in the past: some rocky times but all okay at the moment. I consider the problem being with them and not me: come up blank there.

It's not that I don't know it might be their problem, it's simply that I feel it is probably mine as it has been so many times before. And how often have you asked the person themselves for clarification, only to get a non-committal or brusque reply, which tells you they don't want to talk about it and confirms it most likely was your fault?

By discussing it with someone else, you discover that it *was* you, though not in the way you expected. Your friend reminds you that bringing up the person's past indiscretions may have been relevant to the conversation but that this made them agitated and defensive, which then caused them to take offence at everything you said after.

Hmm, so in this case, the aspie strikes again, brought down once more by the lance of logic, wielded with good grace and even better intentions but without any thought for the bigger picture.

You see how past problems can be ironed out, or at least de-mystified, by examination and a little bit of help? In a similar way, a problem right here and now, in the present, which threatens you with panic or meltdown, can also be resolved by a moment's proper calm or a friendly hand on the shoulder (metaphorically, as the last thing you want to do to an aspie in meltdown is grab them by the shoulder).

The present panic recedes and the day clears again. The moment has passed and the aspie continues on their way, none the worse. So why doesn't this measured response seem to work the next time?

Well, the next time will be completely different, even if it is just the same. Old tactics and logic only work up to a point. Rather like defunct train tracks, you take one that looks very much like another and you are likely to find yourself against the buffers with the right track carrying on without you.

Imagine I have a similar argument to the one I described above. Same person, same responses, same old history to colour the present and the same aspie in the middle of it all, logging the event to dissect it later. A massive stand-off happens, aspie drags emotional self off to a corner and contacts wise friend for a re-cap on what on earth is going on.

The friend suggests this is like the other time, that you said something rotten in the middle of the argument which set everything else in motion. You deny it, you only said the same thing the person has said to you before, except this time it was true for them. This cannot be the same as the other argument because you never said x and it didn't lead to y and it's all totally, completely different.

Wise friend points out it is *almost* the same because you said something better left unsaid in the middle of a heated exchange and then wondered why the other person imploded. You point out, again, this is not the same because last time the thing you said was x and this time it was g: x and g are in no way the same so how can this be compared?

Your friend, now with an edge to their voice, explains that it doesn't matter if you said x or g, **the way the other person felt was the same**. At that stage, I'm left rolling my eyes and waving my hands in the air because, readers, bringing feelings into the thing is what makes this aspie want to leave and live somewhere wild and unpopulated.

So you say x and get y, then you say g and get w and they are meant to be the same because the other person's feelings says they are? Come on! Just when I think I am getting to the bottom of this silly business of facts having different faces depending on who is looking at them, there's another indiscriminate rule I was meant to know without being told.

Is it any wonder I lose my patience and stomp about with steam coming out of my ears? I might as well never speak at all, if this is how it's going to be.

Why not go ahead and just be one big mass of feelings and then I can prod at them, splintering them while you lie there, prostrate in agony? Would that be better?

No, I digress. I do get it, really. I know that other people have their own feelings which can be repeated even when the conversation is different. Yes, it is logical, I will admit it. But why do I have to be responsible? I do all I can, you know. I say what I think is right and am left confused and aghast when I think I have dealt with something the right way and find I have broken it all to pieces yet again.

It makes me feel like not opening my mouth, like standing there in the room, obviously present but inherently absent from what is going on. If feelings can be hurt by a wrong letter then I won't speak at all. Safer to be silent and unyielding than to carry on being the centre of every conversational storm.

Yes, I over-react but so do other people, from my point of view. As an aspie, it is very easy to say the wrong thing, or the right thing at the wrong time, and upset the other person. It is amazingly simple to cause an argument and refresh an old hurt. If only the rest of communication was this doable!

What remains so very, very hard is realising all of these connections while you are in the middle of a conversation and remembering that conversations are linked to who people are and who you are to them. Conversations are never just words, unfortunately. They are living creatures in their own right, stalking the room, looking for prey. They are always waiting for the unwary aspie to tread in and be silhouetted against the setting sun.

Forgive me if I stay in the shadows and avoid the clearing where everyone can see me. Sooner rather than later I know I will hear the oncoming paws, the breath behind, the feeling that I have, yet again, put myself in the wrong place. Sometimes it seems easier to say nothing at all than to bring such drama into life.

Fear of the future

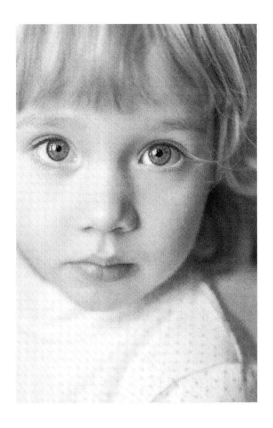

This is a big one for me, a close relation to my need to live in the past and zoom, panicked, through the present. The future can be terrifying to all of us but to an aspie it really is an unknowable country.

You would think, if you were a non-aspie, or a well-meaning best beloved, that the same techniques which work for the past and present might work for the future. Is it not logical to think that by explaining and de-mystifying something, you make it all right?

If the aspie is quaking at the thought of a return to work, knowing it will all go wrong, knowing that quirky feeling they had when they went for the interview is a warning that it is a bad place to be, that the people will be mean or devious or just too loud, that the dress code will never work because they don't suit blue...

If all of this is taking place, even on a small scale, can it not be assuaged by the gentle words, reminding the aspie of all the good things they have to look forward to, that it doesn't matter if they don't suit blue, there will be others who don't suit it, that it's only for three hours a day, that it will all be fine because no one will expect them to know everything when they first start.

Planning ahead, de-constructing the worries, is a very, very important part of Aspergers. Being able to do this keeps me as sane as I'm ever going to be, to imagine what might happen and plan for it. If I start to panic, then I feel I haven't been able to plan enough or, so much worse, **there is nothing I can do to make it better**.

By the time I have started panicking, I've already tried planning and working things out. I've passed the stage of using my own coping mechanisms and am unwilling to consider yours. After all, I know yours don't work for me because we've tried them before and they seem like empty words. I can't *feel* them, not like I can feel mine.

When I plan my first day at work, in the hated blue, I imagine myself walking through the doors and visualise where I will go from there. I worry I won't know which way to go so I visualise someone showing me the right door and the right place to be. I visualise all of this so that I will be able to walk through the door in the first place.

If I am thrown by worry and imagine too many scenarios, or I have the horrible muddy feeling that tells me, no matter what, it's all going to go wrong, then my visualisation will not work properly. I will begin to feel that as I am not coping with the imagined scenarios, there must be one I haven't thought of which will definitely go wrong - how can it go right if I don't foresee it and work out how to deal with it? *That* is logic.

This logic of the aspie, which brings you to a certain point, then leaves you in a primeval fear of the unknown, is what makes future planning very difficult. The scenarios and potential experiences may be different but the response is the same.

It is ahead and it is frightening. If I can't find a way out of the fear, be it real or imagined fear (they become the same thing), then **I will not do it**. It won't matter what you say or do or try, I am steadfast. If you won't protect me from this fear then I'll have to protect myself and that's all there is to it.

I should point out that we aspies are very brave, you know. We feel this fear every day in some way, large or small. It's very often there when you think we're relaxed. You have to be alert always if you know you're in danger and aspies do feel there is constant danger of some kind, lurking round the corner.

So, a fear of the future, the big unknown and therefore the big danger, is bound to make life complicated. This is where lovely routines come in because they're so familiar you don't have to visualise them anymore; they have become a part of you.

It is not hopeless, by any means. As I've said, we're very brave and we will try harder than you expect, even if it doesn't seem very hard from your point of view. It has to be at our own pace, though, and slow enough so that the future doesn't rush at us, too quickly to see it coming and full of sharp things and noise.

Reassurance is key, as is good old patience. We may not listen to your words of comfort - sorry! - but we do listen to the tone and the implicit message that you are there, will always be there, that you love us even when we're hiding behind the sofa, screaming at you.

And sometimes, when the future comes around and happens and wasn't full of sharp things and noise, you can use that as an example to us of how it was all fine in the end and we can do it the next time. Then, visualisation is our friend because we have faced the thing and can imagine facing it again and doing it safely.

Eventually, we may do the new things and be braver than we thought we could be. Sometimes we won't and you'll tear out what little hair you have left trying to get us there. Don't worry, we'll love you even if you're bald (and will ask you if you knew you were bald) and we'll carry on being as aggravating as before, but still ourselves.

In the end, aspies know as well as anyone that the future comes no matter what you do. The trick is in feeling you are ready for it, in small ways, so that it doesn't become too big to cope with. We also know that sometimes the future is massive and can never be managed, even though we have to. That knowledge underlies everything so be patient with us because as you're looking ahead to the small thing we have to do and wondering why we can't do it, we see the very large thing hiding behind it, asking us to face it.

Sometimes we can, but please be patient if we can't.

The aspie effect

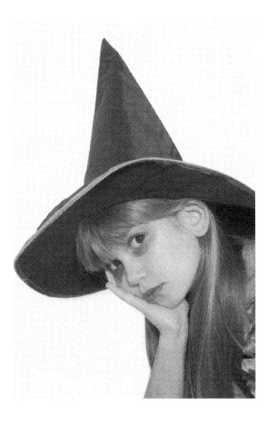

I had one of those moments yesterday, when someone looks at you, looks closer, then seems to try not to flinch backwards. Does that happen to other people too? It always worries me as I think I look quite safe.

I don't wear my special llama hat to go to the shops; I do wear all the items of clothing people usually expect to see. I don't talk to myself when people are close enough to hear, I try to remember not to pull faces when I'm distracted.

Yet sometimes, seemingly through no fault of my own, people behave as if I might attack them, bite, suddenly sing or recite personal anecdotes. I tend to think of it as my witch-effect. It's how I imagine they'd look if I turned out in full regalia - black cloak, cobwebby dress, holey stockings, scary shoes, pointed hat, cat on my shoulder, broom under my arm. *Then* I'd expect people to cringe or change direction.

As it is, I'm what I think of as ordinary. I'm short, I wear glasses, my clothes are usually unremarkable. I'm a woman of a certain age whose hair is possibly reaching the scary stage of long - but surely not scary enough to really scare people?

I do like to wear hobbit-type boots (though before anyone jumps in, yes, I know hobbits don't wear anything on their feet). My bag is an anime-homage that I found on eBay and I sometimes decide it's more important to match colours than styles.

So what? None of this is enough to make people flinch, is it? I do wonder.

Sometimes, small children react this way but it's almost always the adults. I have to say, when it comes to little girls I often have the opposite effect. I've had small girls look up at me and their faces light up as they pass, delighted smiles making me smile in return. I call this the witch-effect too, as most small girls would be excited to see me out with the broom and cat. And no, I haven't got to the bottom of the delighted reaction either.

I think it comes down to one simple reason, for which I don't yet have an explanation: other people see something in me that I don't see in myself.

What could it be? Would it be something I'd want to know about? Could I use it to my advantage? Would knowing make me more self-conscious and less likely to cope? Would it change my life?

Do I simply look different, in a way that is so familiar to me and to people who know me, that none of us sees it anymore? Is it like having a dearly loved aunt with a giant nose: where strangers see a little old lady with massive nostrils, you see the sweet woman who makes life brighter?

Perhaps what I need to do is have someone follow me round and tell me what I do, or film me so I can pick over it obsessively and critique myself on my life skills. No, heavens no, can you imagine? How awful to see yourself that way, to realise how you look to others and then find out there's little you can do to change it. Self-critiquing very quickly turns to self-criticism and we do enough of that already.

I've mostly come to terms with it now. I do like seeing little girls grin up at me as they pass: each time that happens, I feel like I made a new friend. I don't mind so much when people react like I'm a worry. I've come to terms with being different and, if they feel like that, we probably wouldn't be friends anyway, so why bother myself about it?

If I'm perfectly honest, readers (and I wouldn't tell everyone this), I don't mind when people shrink back. I feel that a small, magical part of me has tweaked a tiny, primeval part of them. They suddenly realise that not all people are the same and it worries them.

I just smile a little wider and bend a little closer when it happens, to show them I mean no harm. Of course, this doesn't always assuage their worry but it helps me practice letting people further into my personal space.

I'll allow them the flinch, the step back, the quick frown as they take another look at me. Let them do what they like and maybe, if they look long enough, they'll stop being worried at the difference and notice that I'm smiling at them.

That's when you hope that people see beyond whatever it was that caught their eye to the person beneath. As aspies, we're so often concerned with what goes on under the surface, at the same time as being distracted by what is obvious on the outside. Let other people have the same chance, to see what is obvious, and then to look beneath and see the real you.

If it doesn't work and they don't see you, let it be. Sometimes, it's easier just to smile and talk back to them, pretending you didn't notice their discomfort. You may see them again and get a better reaction. That doesn't matter either.

Readers, what really matters is behaving in the way you would like others to behave towards you. If we keep on smiling, keep on talking and don't use bad reactions as a reason to turn away, then maybe other people will see how we are and carry a little of it with them as they move on.

And if all else fails, just be content with the people whose faces light up as you pass by. They are the ones destined to be your friends, in this place or the next.

What noise?

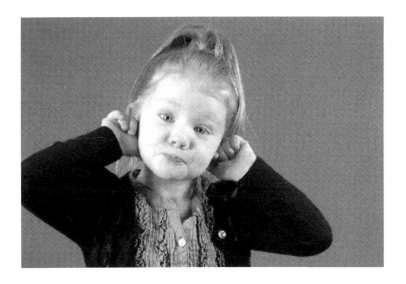

It's a small problem, right? It's not life-threatening: stars will not die nor oceans dry up. The moon will not change in its trajectory across our skies and the world health organisation will not start filling bunkers with nubile examples of the human genome.

It is, after all, only a *noise*.

It's a repetitive, annoying, unstoppable all-assailing noise which has decided to happen near me and cannot be locked out of my head without industrial-grade ear defenders. It is so regular and irritating that I feel as if my head will explode if it doesn't stop.

Anything else I have to do will **stop**. It will grind to a sudden halt as I stand, head on one side, listening to see where the noise is coming from. Once I realise the noise isn't under my control, I am doomed to listen, over and over and over again to this noise which will never end and stretches on forever into what used to be my future.

My teeth ache, caused by the noise. (Okay, possibly caused by setting my jaw in a suffering and rigid position). My head is full of the noise and nothing else stays there for long. Any work I had to do comes second to the noise and any conversations I try to have tail off as I forget what we were saying and listen to the noise.

Other people are often so unaffected by this that I have to explain to them there even *is* a noise and then point out what it is. I stand there, angst-ridden, as they listen and finally hear it. 'Oh yes,' they say and carry on with what they were doing.

Later they might appear and ask, 'Why haven't you made any dinner?'

I look at them as if dinner was some new-fangled idea, then say, 'I was waiting for the noise to stop.'

'What noise?' they ask, having forgotten all about it.

'The noise!' I become animated. 'The noise that's been going on for ages!'

Non-aspies are never going to understand the profound effect of an unfriendly noise on the aspie consciousness. I barely understand it myself

110

as I know, I really, logically know, that a small noise in the distance, or a larger noise next door, will not harm me and shouldn't put a hold on everyday life.

And yet it does. That noise becomes greater than it is, cutting out the aspie's shaky ability to process normal thoughts, making sure that the level of concentration required to hold it all together is disrupted to such an extent that nothing else exists except the noise.

When it stops - bliss... The quiet! It feels like a vacuum, a beautiful emptiness devoid of anything but grace. It is the feeling we all live for, that sense of peace which makes the tumult of life bearable again.

Readers, it has stopped. It has gone. I am close to being human again. Everything denied me for the eternity it lasted is restored. I am whole once more.

4: Disagree?

Disagreements, arguments, difficulties, misunderstandings, they are all part of the aspie universe. Basically, we disagree with many things on principle and are not immune to making life difficult for ourselves. This is a talent, the kind of knack other people do not envy, even if they can admire the scope of our awkwardness.

But we have priorities, you see. Real ones which involve our attention, our whole mind taken up with this aspect of our lives. Being told to leave these priorities behind just because some real-life issue needs out attention seems out of kilter with how things should be. When something is important to us, it takes precedence, no matter if it makes everything complicated further down the line.

Wants and needs are interchangeable and feel the same. I want to know what happens next time on Webs of Hunger and if you expect me to leave the house when it comes on, then I will not be happy. I want to finish the chapter I am writing because if I don't, my mind will separate from it and I will be adrift and it may be a long, long time before I can return to it. The real-life need to send in an important form or visit a relative is secondary – how can it be otherwise with such an essential task ahead of me?

What others see as unnecessary, or at best selfish, I see as vital. I can even explain to you how and why it is vital, but expect me to become agitated if you get that look on your face again. Sometimes it feels like no one will ever understand the creative and inverted to-do list within the aspie consciousness.

This section describes how the aspie priorities butt up against life's necessities, not always making for a happy union. More often it seems to end with the train teetering off the tracks as it makes contact with an unexpected obstacle.

The perfect storm: aspie vs aspie

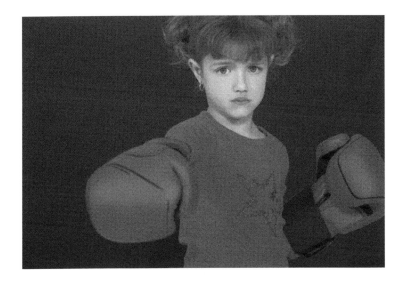

The scene was set for a proper aspie showdown, a chance for all our little niggles to grow and inflate until they take over the house. I asked RT Teen to do something and he messed it up.

Now, if I had swapped those two sentences around, you may have looked at it and thought, 'What's the big deal? Teenagers mess up all the time?' Yes, I know, I am a mother of teenagers and I'm well aware they mess up a lot. As I'm also an aspie, I can't say too much about their messes when I create my own on a daily basis.

RT Teen and I usually get along very well, both in our haze of aspie-ness, buffered from the real world by the belief that our inner lives are as important as the outer. Sometimes we crash up against each other (and sometimes that's literally, if we both rush for the same door), but usually we're happy to accept each other for who we are.

When we do collide, it's nearly always on a grand scale, often set off by me not watching how I say something so that RT takes an instant, no-return-policy kind of offence and flounces up the stairs, the house shaking around him. Or, sometimes, it's me who loses it...

I've done my best, readers. I try to not fly off the handle and fall foul of my aspie nature when I'm also being a mother. I admit my obsessive traits and irresponsible nature. I struggle to be an adult for as long as I can, then hide in a corner and hope no one needs me until I recharge. But I am only human.

On this particular day, as with most dramas, it started quietly. We had the shopping delivered from Asda, my new way of saving money. Ordering online stops me going in all the time and wandering. It's like a magic trick, making my money go further just by keeping me away from the shop.

IT Teen had to call in at college, so we waited for the shopping then left, with me telling RT to put away the frozen and chilled food. Simple, right? (I can hear those who have parented teenagers sighing at this point).

116

While we were out, RT called me. I thought someone had died, honestly. He said, in the darkest, saddest, slowest of voices, 'Um, erm, oh...' dramatic pause, 'the mouse has completely broken. It won't work at all! Can you get one while you're out?'

Panic averted, IT and I went to find a mouse. Like anything IT buys, there has to be a prolonged investigation into the merits and geek value of any item, with some internet reviews to back it up. A triumph for modern parenting, I managed to come away with the cheapest one on the shelf.

Finally, after an hour and a quarter we came home. There, waiting to greet us, was the shopping. No, not all of it, he'd put away the orange juice. Yes, hmm. And the fish fingers. The rest of his time had been spent discovering the mouse had broken, then discovering if he pressed the mouse hard enough it still worked and then doing his art on Gimp.

All this time the shopping had sat in our summer-warm hallway, gently defrosting, warming or rotting, depending on its nature. I saw red.

There was commotion, involving flailing of arms, battle cries, much pointing at bags and IT (uncharacteristically) vanishing to his room. Our dogs even left us to it. The cats, ever hopeful, circled the bag of ex-fish we had been going to have for tea.

After much natural expression, RT started to put away what was left of the shopping. As he stocked the fridge, the new packet of mini pies fell out, opening on the way down and tumbling all over the floor. At this point, I

117

saw ultraviolet. Before I could deconstruct in the middle of the kitchen, I stalked off to the living room, saying, 'I'm going to be on my own for a while...'

As I hadn't said, 'leave me alone,' RT followed me ten seconds later to say he'd put all the frozen and chilled away. The young dog started vibrating in his bed, expecting us to turn into fireworks again. This part of the fiasco was not helped by RT entering the self-pity stage of the row earlier than was safe.

He wanted my sympathy as he'd had a bad few days where he kept forgetting things. He couldn't remember what he'd forgotten, but he knew he had and he was sad about it. You can imagine how sympathetic I was. There were a few more rockets set off then he retreated to his room.

I cooked our ex-fish for cat supper instead of ours, forgetting about it as it cooked and wondering what strange things they had on the barbeque next door. The cats were very glad of the fish and made me feel a little better about having to eat something else.

I then turned the fridge up as it seemed to have got a bit warm and I didn't want to lose even more food. After this, RT and I made friends, with him acknowledging responsibility for the cats' supper and me nit-picking over what I had done and said to see if I could have been any more patient (I could, but then I'd have been a Stepford mother).

There are two post scripts to this story. One is that IT and I won't be putting away any shopping for a very long time. The other is that I don't know which way is ON for the fridge temperature control. I had turned it down instead of up and was back at Asda yesterday morning, replacing yoghurts and the like, having fed our very, very happy cats on cooked pork and cheese.

It did work out in the end and we came back to our stable understanding with barely a whiff of 'I told you so' from IT Teen (he knows when to shut up sometimes). We also have very contented cats who are almost crazed when I come in with a shopping bag now. That's going to make life difficult for a while.

Other than that, it's all normal aspie stuff, I guess. The kind of thing you find hard to explain to other people but, at the time, you think to yourself, 'This is why life is never going to be boring'.

I'm an aspie not a Star Fleet captain

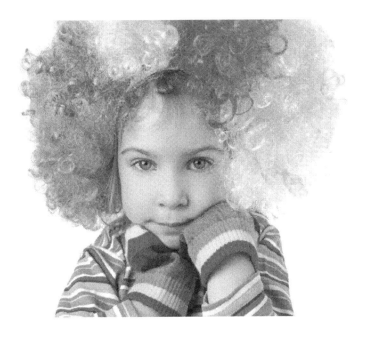

Aspergers, it's just so selfish and demanding. Whatever you want to do, it has to come first.

You wanted to be a high-powered business person? Go on then, try it with Aspergers running ahead and kicking people up the butt while you're not looking. A surgeon or a fire-fighter? Same thing; Aspergers pushes ahead, trying to put you off, no matter what you do.

Scale it back and all you want to do is get ready for your exams or an important job interview. Cue Aspergers, bustling in at the door, acting like it knows best, making it seem like a great idea to concentrate on only *this* part of your upcoming event and not look at the whole thing.

Or perhaps Aspergers clashes the cymbals and bangs the drum so you can't concentrate on anything at all? That's worse as you know exactly what you have to do and can't make your brain work long enough to get it done.

Scale it back again and all you have to remember is to pick up your mother from the train station. Aspergers lives for moments like these because they come along more often than the massive job interviews or life-changing career decisions.

Somehow, while you're not looking, Aspergers sneaks in and puts the kettle on, letting you get settled with your tea, looking at your emails and ordering that set of Star Trek figurines on eBay. Great news! You won them and at a fraction of the price. You can't wait to have them set out in the space you already made in the bedroom.

Bad news: that annoying noise in the background, the one that kept interrupting the eBay auction, was your mobile phone on vibrate. Your mother is also vibrating, much more loudly, on the freezing cold steps of the train station. While you got on with your important work, she watched the other commuters hurry home or get picked up. One by one they left until it's only her, waiting for you, as usual.

It's no good apologising, then trying to make it better by telling her about the figurines. It doesn't even work if you tell her about the figurines as if it all happened on another day. She will *know*. She'll know that you spent the time bidding on eBay instead of collecting her from the cold station. She'll know that the figurines were more important to you than your own mother. Yet again, she'll despair of you.

Yes, all of these lifestyle complications are caused by Aspergers, that jester at the feast, that syndrome with the sense of humour only a fool could find funny.

Aspergers as a great distractor is well-known - ask anyone who has had to live with an aspie for very long. But Aspergers as the saboteur may not be so familiar, at least to the outside world.

I think this is because, as aspies, it's easier to explain to people that having Aspergers makes you forget things more easily or become distracted or simply focus too much on the wrong thing. All of these are true and simple to imagine.

It's much more difficult to explain the idea of Aspergers helping you to self-destruct. And here, I can't put all the blame on Aspergers, as if it's an annoying uncle who thinks it's funny to poke you in the ribs when you take a drink. It can be like that but when Aspergers enters the sabotage mode, it always needs an accomplice.

I can honestly say I didn't know that myself and Aspergers were saboteurs until a few years ago. It's a surprise to discover that so many of your misadventures were helped along by your own willingness to participate, or even instigate, events that cause everything around them to collapse.

It's a hard thing to admit, that you could have achieved more and done better if you had only ignored some of your impulses and gone on as planned. The number of times I've seen something good on the horizon - and fill in whatever positive life event you like here - and then found myself working against it.

A simple example would be that all-important interview. You need the job, the money and, more to the point, would *like* the job itself. What do you do? Well, you know what you're wearing but don't check it's all okay beforehand. You know what time you have to be there but don't give yourself the extra half hour to get ready. You know you need to look your best but decide to leave washing your hair until the morning.

Anything and everything can be scattered in the path of success. You only need to stand on one sharp tack to stumble and fall; with Aspergers you can guarantee you'll throw a few more down, just to be sure.

Assuming you make it past all these obstacles and get to the interview on time, it still won't be what it promised because you're now flustered at having to fight to be there. The answers you might have given are subtly changed, lessened by the distraction of the morning's events. You're not looking quite as smooth as you should and you forgot to polish your shoes.

Now, I don't know if any of you are grumbling about it yet, but don't worry, I haven't forgotten about the aspies who find their niche and become brilliant successes. I haven't, honestly. Where do they fit in to this scenario of the sneaky Aspergers making things go wrong? Surely they have no place as the self-saboteur?

I believe there is only the barest, most subtle difference between these successful people and the aspie toddling along with mismatched shoelaces. The successful aspie recognised Aspergers for what it was years before the rest of us even realised it existed. They saw that they were different and they factored it into their lives. They also never lost their self-belief.

How did they do this? What is their secret? Each one would have a different story. I think it lies in them having a more positive view of themselves which then made them see their talents in a good way too.

If you believe you are a good and worthy person, it's much more likely that you want to share your talents with the outside world. You believe in yourself therefore you believe in your talents too.

It doesn't have to be this simple but if Aspergers can be spotted creeping in and if you have the self-confidence, you can quickly jump up and slam the door so it can't get all the way through. Better still, let Aspergers creep in then jump up and offer it a seat. Make it part of the equation.

How you do this is a pickle, to say the least. Again, it's different for everyone. I think it's brilliant if you can bring up your little aspies to think this way. If young Tommy can't get his ideas down onto paper, don't study the textbooks or consult specialist teachers for ways to pry the information from his brains. Take him out to play in the leaves instead. If that information needs to come out, then it will, but only when he can let it pass.

Build up little Tommy's confidence and self-belief, let him see his aspie traits as a difference and not a disability. Let him know that you're there to help and not to push. Tell him it will all be okay in the end, that you love him and he loves you and it's a good day for a walk in the park.

If you're an older aspie, only now realising that you're up to your eyeballs in sharp tacks, take a step back and have a big, ponderous think. You know you love doing that. But this time, think about your role in life in a different way. Don't use the F word (failure), consider things in new ways.

What did you really do when the money ran out? Were you really being stupid and irresponsible? Possibly, but were you also thumbing your nose at the world and saying, 'I can spend it if I want! No one is telling *me* what to do!'?

Look at your motivations - the ones that power you to behave in a certain way. It may be the Aspergers at work, it may not. Sometimes, it could be *you* at work, making sure you're not set up to fail again by stopping things in their tracks before they go too far towards success.

There is no magic solution for side-stepping the difficulties caused by Aspergers and fulfilling your potential. This is one of those areas where other people can play as pivotal a role as you do. For young aspies, it is essential to help them gain self-confidence and inner happiness. For older aspies, working it out for themselves is more important because the defensive structures are already in place and they won't be as ready to believe what other people say to boost them up.

Be self-aware. See what happens and why, even if you have to go away and work it all out later. Even if later is years down the line, still take the time to work it out.

And believe me, I'm not saying aspies can't do any and all of the jobs they want - it just may take a different route to get there and a little more care along the way.

We all need a clear view to see where we're going, otherwise we'll keep wandering into the same dead ends and side alleys, bumping over the pot-holes as we go. Take your time and think about what happened the last time and what you really want to happen now.

It could be that you're telling yourself you don't want this high-powered job interview, that what you really want is to get out the old guitar and re-visit a time when the music flowed unbidden into the world.

You see, Aspergers isn't just a jester or a saboteur. Aspergers knows us *so well* and it remembers the music of our childhood when anything was possible and the world didn't seem as big. Sometimes, you need to read between the lines and see what it is you're trying to tell yourself.

This is how you find the right road.

Aspies have things they need to do

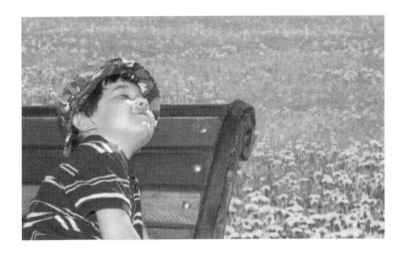

Aspies can be very problematic, either in a specific way, such as panicking in crowded places, or a more general way, like those days when they will not leave the warm glow of the computer, no matter what.

If a best beloved needs to go out shopping and their aspie must come too, then the specific problem of crowded places plus the generalised annoyance of the aspie basking in the computer's ambience, both have a grounding effect. The best beloved must take their aspie out but the aspie is determined to stay at home.

This is where conflict begins, no matter how patient the best beloved might be. That moment when they realise the aspie has dug in their heels and wants to stay put.

It begins warmly, with encouragement: they need to go out, this needs to be done and everything will be fine. The aspie hears 'need' and automatically discounts it: the aspie really needs to stay here and wait for the next episode of Webs of Hunger to be released onto YouTube.

The outing needs to take place, it is necessary, it must be done sometime. The encouragement has turned into cajoling organisation, trying to make it seem as if there is no choice. Sooner or later, the aspie will be leaving the house.

Aspie hears the 'sometime' and 'sooner or later'. This kind of phrasing often by-passes a whole conversation and is the only part which sticks. If the job can be done sometime or sooner or later, then why not later? Why do these jobs always need done sooner? Where is the logic in that?

After all, Webs of Hunger will be ready to watch sooner not later and in the next half an hour not sometime. Logic would dictate that Webs of Hunger is far more important than this vague need to do unnecessary jobs in a crowded shopping place.

And anyway, why does the aspie have to come?

At this point, best beloved is forced to reveal that the aspie will be clothes shopping, for *themselves*. This is the part of the conversation where arms start to jig and lips contort and eyes flare like a Klingon faced with social niceties.

After a pause for a lot of words which amount to the aspie needing new clothes and those clothes needing to fit and the whole modern world being built around the necessity of not going to your cousin's wedding wearing a suit from 1985, the aspie reluctantly concedes that new clothes will have to be bought,

Later, though.

Best beloved is faced with the aspie's back, hurriedly turned, their hand over the mouse, fingers quivering in expectation of the page refreshing and revealing Webs of Hunger, Episode 6, where we finally discover if Chartra is alive or has been fed, piece by piece, to Halendra's children.

Knowing this battle is lost, best beloved does what best beloveds often do in this situation and puts the kettle on, then calls a close friend. It's either that or scream in the middle of the garden. Or unplug the internet and run away with the hub (but look how that turned out last time).

Sooner or later, the aspie will be dragged from the house to the department store and clothes will be bought. Crowds will be endured and changing rooms will be used for great lengths of time, disproportionate to the amount of clothes taken into them.

Best beloved will watch at the changing room door, mulling over the possibility of measuring every part of the aspie's body so that clothes can be bought with a tape measure in tow instead of a great heap of reluctant aspie.

Sooner or later, the cousin's wedding will loom too, a bigger feat of endurance than any shopping trip and filled with many small dramas and interesting situations. But throughout it all, best beloved will be secure in the knowledge that whatever happens to the custard pie, their aspie looks great in the new clothes and they won't have to go shopping again for a very long time.

The inner conversation

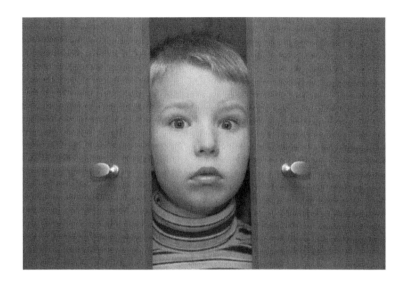

"When the time comes I can have the connection on this part and then I can see what works because the last time I tried it, it didn't work and I had to wait four hours to get back online. That was a drag because I wanted to be online and-"

What did you want for tea?

"…and I thought it might be permanent or that I'd have to pay to have it fixed which would be terrible. The last time I paid to have anything fixed-"

I asked what you wanted for tea?

…

What do you want?

I'm not hungry

"So, I could wait until I'm sure then ask Gen what to do as he knows how to work it round the right way and he never seems to lose connection-"

What??!

You have to eat something! I've got some oat cakes and then there's the pizza from yesterday and the-

"Gen, I was going to ask him, oh, what was I thinking? I had it all worked out!"

-orange juice as well, which is quite nice or I could-

"It was in this file, I think, I'm sure I put it in an easy place and, ah, that's the old one. Hang on, it's probably on a different-"

Well?

Well, what?!

There's no need for that tone of voice! I'm waiting to see what you want for tea.

I said I wasn't hungry! I'm trying to concentrate!

You're only on the computer, I'm sure you could spare me five seconds to say what you want to eat.

I don't want to eat! I'm not just on the computer! I'm working!!

You're only doing what you always do, waiting for your friends to come online. That isn't work, you know. Work is when people go out to do jobs for a living or what I have to do, every day, while you sit there doing goodness knows what online.

It is work! I am working! You have no idea! I do not want to eat or drink anything and if I did I could get it for myself!!!

Fine! Just fine! Get it yourself then, see if I care! (sob)

"Where was I? What time is it? Why do people always want me to talk to them? I can't even remember what I was doing now. I'll have to start from the beginning.

If only I could have enough peace and quiet, I would get everything done.

Now, let me check this and then I can work that round to-

Hmm, my stomach kind of aches. I wonder if I'm hungry?"

Communicating under pressure

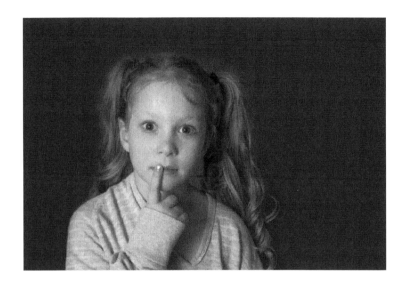

The frustrating thing about talking to your aspie is that you are part of a much bigger picture, but you can only see part of it. To the non-aspie the conversation is between two people and whatever the difficulties, there is no real, proper reason why the words should not pass and be understood. To the aspie, there is so much more going on.

On a good day, the aspie might be distracted, thinking about other things - nothing important but certainly something more interesting than the non-aspie's obsession with getting out of the house by 10am. There are always *lots* more important things than leaving by 10am and they all take precedence in the aspie's wonderfully-ordered mind. So it is that the memory of dropping biscuits into the cow field at the age of five easily pushes aside the droning about being late again.

On a middling day, which covers many days, the aspie is not only distracted by the wonderfully-ordered mind but also by the ticking sound the cooker makes when you forget to knock it off or the way the curtains blow in the wind as you insist on opening the windows. Or the sound of next-door's car alarm going off yet again because it is impossible for a grown adult, supposedly an advanced species, to remember to switch off the alarm before they use the key.

A middling day may be full of many nuisances which do nothing to harm the aspie but have the power to drive them into ditches, over and over, right through the day.

Meanwhile, the non-aspie is trying to talk to their aspie about the documents they had through the post yesterday, the ones put in a safe place so they could be used today. Firstly, you assume your aspie remembered to put them in a safe place; then you assume your aspie considers them important - properly important, not just important to you and the rest of the world.

You forget that the car alarm has set off *again* and how many times does a person need to open and shut the doors of a car before they get in and drive away?! What documents? What are you talking about? Can't you see your aspie is stressed? What do you mean there's nothing to be stressed about?

You're always wanting something and everything is so difficult! (Cue melodramatic exit to place of safety).

Then there are the bad times. Luckily, these don't often last a day, they just feel like they do. These are the times when the bigger picture is full of dangers and trials, overflowing with awful endeavours all sent to push your aspie right into their mini-breakdown and out of the reach of anyone, even you.

To the non-aspie, it is a place somewhere, an everyday place. People go there all the time. It could be a busy shop, a hospital, a friend's party (see, it's safe because it's a *friend's* party), a street full of shoppers (see, it's safe because we don't have to go *inside* the shops), the school at home-time, the college at going-in time - anywhere that has enough triggers or big enough stresses to make your aspie feel the world has come to an end and is now broken into many loud, dangerous, floating pieces of life which defy understanding.

Amidst all this life-threatening chaos, you want to talk to your aspie and have them listen? You want to ask them something? You want a conversation? Would you have a conversation in the middle of a war-zone? If soul-stretching demons were descending, would you want to talk then? If you were in the primeval forest and a soft breathing sound came from behind, would you pause to discuss the weather and then get tetchy when your aspie acted as if you were mad?

I know, it is drama. It reads like your aspie is constantly over-reacting. But it is only over-reacting if you are not the person living through it. A fear is only groundless if you are not the one in the grip of it. A drama is only divorced from real-life if your life is not full of drama already. A conversation only makes sense if both people are able to have it, at the same time.

And just because you can't see the bigger picture doesn't mean it isn't there.

Sometimes it is a very big picture and your aspie a small speck amongst it. Other times the picture is contracting and doesn't leave enough space for life. Try to see how complicated a conversation can become under these conditions and then be kind to your aspie.

A Proper Aspie

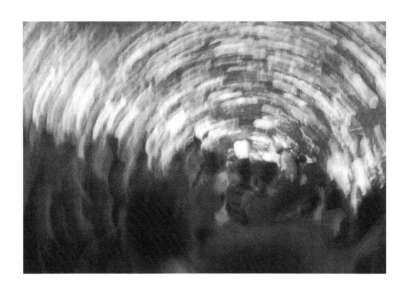

Are you a proper aspie? Do people you know treat you as an aspie? Do they discuss *your* Aspergers, as opposed to Aspergers in general? Or are you the person who forgot to pay the phone bill long enough for it to be shut off because who needs a landline anymore and now you realise the internet comes through the landline and you have to pay through the nose to get it all connected again?

The truth is, aspies are all these things: the term Aspergers covers so much, a literal spectrum of behaviours, traits, modes of thought, difficulties, genius ideas and creativity. The other truth is that aspies are people who make mistakes and also make history. Somewhere in between is where your family and friends place you.

141

In some families, aspies are treated differently because of their Aspergers, more carefully or in a particularly sensitive way. Mostly these are families with child or teen aspies. Those of us who grew to be off-the-wall adults are usually treated as off-the-wall adults, not aspies. (There are exceptions, of course, but most people who contact me online are adults who grew up before Aspergers was recognised).

For me as the off the wall/aspie adult, it doesn't seem to matter if there have been in-depth, personal conversations about what Aspergers means, I am still a screw-up when I get it wrong. Yes, I have problems but who doesn't? Other people manage.

And if Aspergers rears its head, it is dismissed, seen as a word to cover faults or an excuse to get out of trouble. This is not said outright but it is felt. After all, if Aspergers is to blame for the whole phone line fiasco, then it stops me being in trouble, right?

Wrong. I don't expect to get out of trouble and I don't expect to be unaccountable for all the times I break life. What I would like is to be seen as an individual who does not do these things just because I feel like it. I am not avoiding responsibility and by-passing important choices because I am a flake; I am behaving in a way dictated by how I feel and how much I can cope with.

I might seem like a flake when I let people down and forget what I promised to do but if I could explain it to you, in a comforting sequence of events, I could show you how Monday led to Tuesday and by Wednesday I was ready for Saturday. And it would not help to have it pointed out that everyone longs for Saturday.

I do not want to sound like I'm putting myself or other aspies on a pedestal. I am stating a fact when I say, we are not like other people. It's just that, a simple fact. Sometimes we know we have jumped ship, other times we are too busy treading water to realise we're sinking. And all the while we are looking at you, watching your reaction, judging when it is best to jump in and try to do what is right.

There is so much to consider. Other people are simply a part of the grand landscape of life, teeming with ideas and events and objects and feelings, busily vying for our attention; in the midst of this we are trying to focus on the right way to move through. One small thing is easily missed and so is a big thing. When you are surrounded by chaos, small and big no longer matter in the way they do to other people. They become part of the blur of activity, happening on the outskirts of your mind, trying to break in and make you part of the chaos.

Enough! I push it away and disengage and that's the best part of any process. I draw back and separate, I reclaim that central, peaceful part of me which helps me move through the confusion. And somehow, amongst all of these life-changing emotions, I try to remember the silly details of a normal life.

I cope, I step, I talk, I declare myself free of this and one who can move forward and not be dragged from the path. I will leave it to one side and then-

And then I am rediscovered and told I have to behave and cope with events which mean nothing to me. I am trying to save my life and yet I'm supposed to hesitate long enough to pay a bill? How is that logical?

Life is not logical but I keep trying to make it so. Other aspies, proper aspies who have people looking after them and who feature on TV programmes, they are shown as being separate and different. They have their own lives and they do what they can. I am different from them because we are all unique: Aspergers loves the unique.

A proper aspie is every person with Aspergers, whether they lead quiet lives gently guided by others or are on the top of their heap, obsessively downloading sales reports. We are all proper and we all find ourselves on the same path with a whirligig of life jumbling past.

Didn't you think of that before?!

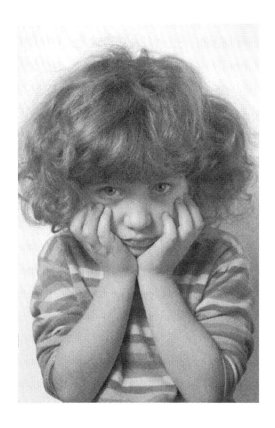

How many times have I been asked this question? I expect it's a question most aspies are familiar with. You do something and before you know it - wham! it's gone wrong and there is always someone willing to pop up and say, 'Didn't you think of that before?'

The situation is irrelevant, as is the calamity which ensues. It is the implied criticism which stings the most once it's all over. No, of course you didn't consider the full consequences of your actions. If you had, would we all be standing here in the ruins of yet another plan?

Ahem. Well, if we're completely honest, we might admit that we did think a little bit of it could go wrong. But that doesn't mean we expected the pitfall to actually *happen*. We might have been able to take into account that it might; we just never thought it would. Do you see the difference?

With the kind of aspie mind-control we seem to believe we possess, we looked into the future and saw the whole thing as a glorious success. Like Picard, we only needed to raise our finger and say, 'Make it so!' for it to succeed. It always slips our minds that smooth runnings generally happen to other people, not to mention the fact that Picard had as many takes as he needed to get everything right first time.

In unguarded moments, I have admitted to deciding to risk it, despite foreseeing possible mishaps. Oh dear, what a mistake that always is! Cue the eye-rolling, the hand-flapping, the exaggerated body language. No, not from the aspie, you understand, but from whichever trusted person we were honest with.

What started as generalised and implied criticism over how things have turned out becomes very specific criticism, mixed with stage-subtle disbelief when we admit we foresaw trouble and jumped regardless.

It seems that admitting you may have been wrong is an open invitation to be jumped up and down on by people who think you should have known better. It's aspie open season at Calamity Acres.

After all, if you saw it coming, why did you carry on? What madness possessed you? What is the point of having that quirkily intelligent head on your shoulders if all you do with it is nod sorrowfully when things go wrong? Did it not occur to you to stop before it was too late?

If I was honest, and if you were honest, we would admit that yes, we saw it coming. Yes, we saw the disadvantages. Yes, we saw the possible calamity awaiting us. And yes, despite all of that, we did it anyway. And no, we aren't completely mad, we just thought it would be okay. Why? Well, because we *hoped* it would be and we could imagine it being okay, so logically it probably was going to be okay.

Non-aspies might be grimly familiar with this scenario, wondering how we don't learn from our past mistakes. Things go wrong so frequently, it defies belief that we'd be willing to get it wrong again and often on a grand scale. Then we have the temerity to take exception to a little bit of criticism! I mean, it's the non-aspies and best beloveds who have to sort it all out once we've finished making our magic; they are entitled to a small dig, aren't they?

Humph. Maybe, maybe not. I don't know about the rest of you aspies but I do hate that people feel they have the right to point out our failings. It's not as if we don't know about them, is it? And at least we have a go, you know, instead of just playing it safe all the time. The told-you-so brigade are not usually the most adventurous souls!

No, let's face it, the real reason we can't take this (often justified) criticism is because we know we are wrong. There, I've said it. You are right and we are wrong. We did it again.

This time, though, it might have been different. It might have worked out and a great and new and wondrous thing would have been let loose across the earth, for all to see and feel uplifted by. Or at the very least, the toilet might have stayed unblocked long enough for the bathroom to be safe.

We try, you see. Again and again, we try and hope that it will turn out all right. Our ideas may be off course and strangely skewed, but they're pretty fabulous ideas half the time. You have to admit, if it had worked, it would have been great!

Just remember, aspie and non-aspie, that we don't do these things to make life horrible or awkward. And we certainly don't do them so we can have someone stand at our shoulder, tutting.

We do them because sometimes they do work and someday we will set the world alight. We just have to keep trying and this means thinking of the consequences and doing it anyway.

5: Aspies in control?

Yes, we can be right and we can be in charge and woe betide the person who stands in our way when we feel like this! Aspies often suffer from low elf-esteem and anxiety so that being in charge of anything only feels like extra stress. However, when we think we are right, such pressures fall away and we have confidence.

Unfortunately, this often translates to the kind of confidence which allows no interference or criticism. From one extreme to another, we move from being awash in life's outer tributaries, to being in the very centre of what is going on. We know this! We can do this! Why isn't everyone doing this?!

We become bossy, opinionated, so sure of our rightness that everything else becomes a wrongness. We are the ones who know the right and true way to do what needs to be done and it is only logical that you will listen, because we know…

It isn't always this extreme but the strength of feeling goes some way to explain why aspies might appear rigorously stubborn in the face of what you or others need them to do. If an aspie thinks they know what is correct, nothing will change that belief. And it can lead to a lot of upset and stress if they are then forced to change what they are doing and do things the 'wrong' way.

This section does not only talk about aspies in the right, it also covers other areas where aspies behave differently from an expected role. I wanted to show that we are all uniquely individual, in ways that surprise our best beloveds or society at large.

The lecturing aspie

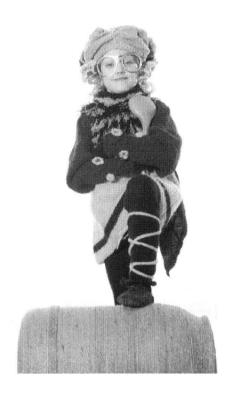

We've all been there: you say something offhand or ask a question and away they go! The aspie who lectures is avoided second only to the aspie who loves to share their obsessions.

Many non-aspies think this tendency to lecture people is a part of being an obsessive aspie - it comes across that way, after all. To the outsider, the aspie in mid-lecture looks very much like the aspie in mid-obsessive monologue. There is the same bright gleam in the eye, the same body language, often the same mannerisms, all designed to make the listener pay greater attention and go away converted.

It might surprise you to know that aspies who give lectures are actually far removed from just sharing their obsessions. The differences between an obsessive monologue and an informative lecture are apparent if you look at the intention behind them.

The aspie who wants to share their obsession truly wants to convert you. They don't want to just tell you about their great love and its many wonders; they want *you* to love it too, at least as much as they do. There is a fervent expectation running through the aspie's whole being as they share everything they know about their pet subject.

The aspie who lectures you does so for your own good, to help you or to save you from something. The subject of the lecture will be close to the aspie's heart, possibly from hard experience or an in-depth knowledge. They want to help you avoid mistakes and succeed.

The fact that a lecture and an obsession can come across as the same thing is a source of frustration in the aspie world. Imagine you give a talk on fire safety, knowing it could save the lives of your audience. And then imagine giving the talk while your audience tries to get away, talks over you, checks their phone, changes the subject or suddenly sees someone they know and leaves.

How would you feel, knowing you were telling them something important only to have them behave as if you were some mad bloke they met on the bus? It isn't good, is it, to have important information treated in the same way as an easily-dismissed obsession?

The aspie is seen as an inconvenience at times, to be humoured and guided away from their troublesome pet subjects. We know how it is. However taken up we are with sharing our obsession, we can still tell when you're trying to get away or not really listening. We simply can't resist the temptation to keep on trying until you see things as we do.

It is far worse, though, to have something important to share and be treated in the same way as always. Do you not even listen to the first sentence? Do you switch off as soon as we start to speak? Or is it the subtle change in our body language that sends you running?

I've had the experience many times of trying to give someone information that could save them a whole load of trouble - money, hard-earned time, even heartache and sorrow - only to be dismissed or humoured as if I was a five year old explaining how butterflies come from caterpillars.

Worse, sometimes the information is treated with derision or impatience, as if what I have to say cannot matter because it comes from me.

I've reached the stage where, with certain people, I hold my peace and let them get on with it. I know I can help them, give them at least part of the key to solving their problems or advancing more quickly. But you do get tired of being ignored, you know?

So, don't be too quick to vacate the room if you meet the lecturing aspie. We might not be at our most scintillating in lecture-mode - it is possibly one of our most boring settings - but if you stick around and listen, you might find out something useful.

And like all good lectures, you should at least look as if you're paying attention because we *will* be asking questions afterwards.

Do as your aspie tells you

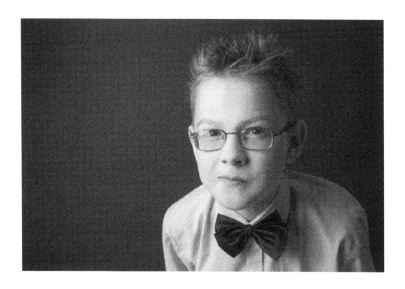

Look, I've been through this plenty of times. Why won't you do what I tell you? Why do you insist on not doing it the right way? I know I get things wrong sometimes but I know best this time. Why won't you listen?

It's really frustrating to be able to see a clear way for someone you care about to make life better and then be ignored. And so, because you care and because you know you have it right, you push on. Determined to make them do what is best, *nothing* will stand in your way.

Whatever it takes, readers, is what an aspie will do when they know best. There is no obstacle big enough to put off the bossy aspie who has the solution right there, ready to use. Your nearest and dearest will take your advice, why wouldn't they? And if they seem a little hesitant, then that hesitancy must be blown away like a cobweb and the helpfulness slotted in its place.

The logic of the aspie argument is undeniable and so the help is also undeniable. It is logical to help yourself, it is logical to follow the aspie plan, there is no other way to do things as the other ways are not logical. And you have so far failed to help yourself or resolve your problems, so even if you can't see the logic in the aspie plan, where is the harm in trying it?

The incessant dripping of this logic can be heard for miles around. It is unstoppable, filling every gap in consciousness, exposing faults and weaknesses, uncovering the fault lines in relationships and making emails and texts a battle ground of evocative, dynamic, unyielding discussions.

Best beloveds will feel sandblasted by the constant barrage of logic and help and persuasion and discussion and argument and why won't you do as I say? It is a stubborn individual who can withstand the aspie in full flow. Aspies may make a lot of mistakes but when they have the solution, there can be only one.

Do as you are told and your life will improve; do as I say and all will be well; do as I plan and it will come together; do this and that will happen. There is no room for failure or missed opportunities. This will work. Logic prevails and best beloveds will be helped and the aspie has no doubt whatsoever.

No doubt at all. Look at those words. When the aspie is sure they can help and sure they have the right method then there is no doubt. And can you imagine how frustrating it is to have no doubt at all and then be faced with the illogical, ridiculous situation of the other person not taking your advice? Crazy!

So we try again from a different angle, except it is the same angle and we come up against the hard fortress of your will with the grappling hooks and flying monkeys of our ideas. There will be a battle, there may be a siege. People will get hurt. And eventually, one way or the other, the walls will come down.

It is not that the aspie is right (even though they are); it is the idea itself which is right. The idea has become an unassailable concept, full of surety and without error. This idea will resolve that problem. Use the idea and help yourself.

Use it, the idea is logical, there is no sense in resisting. There is no way it could go wrong. Did you not understand me? Did I not explain it well enough? Shall I explain it again?

Aspies have no sense of humour

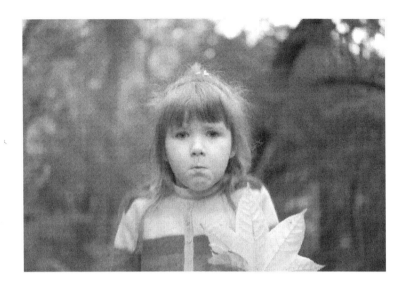

Cough. Hmm. This is one of those statements that brings out the worst in me. On a good day, it just makes me want to kick the person, or get some big, butch bloke to kick the person for me, depending how incensed I'm feeling (I have small feet, kicking doesn't always do the trick).

On a bad day, though, the idea that aspies have no sense of humour makes me feel most rebellious and I want to behave inappropriately. I don't usually streak down the street, scream at dog-walkers, chase the tyres of moving cars or eat all the candy in the Christmas aisle. No, what I do is lose verbal (or typal) inhibitions and let loose the humour-geese.

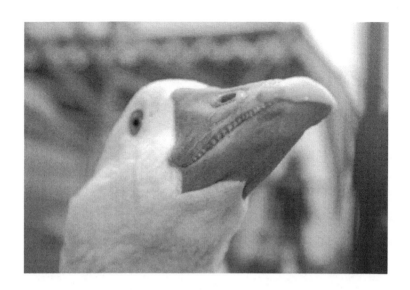

You may not have heard of the humour-geese. I was surprised by them myself. It's what I call my inadvisable moments, when I rise to the challenge of a humourless situation and **funny-it-up**. I can't often resist this challenge. I would say it's like a red rag to a bull but bulls have no choice in the matter and I do. I choose to be funny when I shouldn't.

It's not just for those situations where people make statements about Aspergers - as I've been under-cover for most of my life, they only occasionally say these things to me. More likely, they'll have talked about my son and *his* Aspergers. The sense of humour **jibe** (let's call it what it is) sometimes came up when he was younger, as part of the diagnostic process. It was killed where it stood by my son finding something funny and laughing infectiously until only Cruella de Vil could have resisted joining in.

For myself, I come from a witty, if sometimes cutting, family and have always seen the funny side of things. I like all kinds of comedy on TV, I read funny books, I make jokes, can laugh at myself and others and see the funny side at the least beneficial moments. I've even had to sneak off to the toilets before now to cry with laughter so that I could return without danger of laughing out loud.

I have to add, in case I sound like a hysterical loon at this point, that I also laugh a lot on the inside, at those little moments in life where you find something riotous but can keep it in. I love those. They're often subtle, hard to relate moments, where you are in the right time and place to witness true humour.

I do have to say, if I hadn't been so shy all my life, my sense of humour would have got me into a lot more trouble than it has. Thankfully, nerves often prevent me from blurting out the hilarious thing taking place inside my head so that people are instead faced with me doing a weird little smile as I see the funny side of my unspoken joke at the same time as trying to listen to what they have to say.

My irascible Granda, who often accused me of laughing at him (not just me, he thought *everyone* was laughing at him), might have been forgiven sometimes for thinking I actually was, as I'd drift away from his chuntering and think of other things. If I saw the funny side of my own thoughts then I was in trouble, as he was the master at looking up at the right moment to catch the change in my expression.

Then you're faced with the choice between explaining what you thought was funny, or denying anything was funny. As your own thoughts are just that and it would be hard to translate them, I always opted for denial. This adds to the general reputation you have for not telling the truth because you're obviously *not* telling the truth, you just don't want to share.

The real answer, when caught having a laugh to yourself, is to say you thought of something funny and don't want to share it. This seems so much worse than the other two though, as you sound more mysterious and secretive than ever. We really cannot win.

I've also heard that aspies are allowed to have a sense of humour but that they need the jokes to be obvious and self-explanatory. Jokes written with crayons perhaps? Or coloured in by five year olds?

I wonder about this. Life is full of unusual subtleties that aspies grasp for and miss. Jokes can be the same but I believe we fare better here than in other areas. In my mind, I'm so into humour that I'm on the lookout for it. Perhaps that makes me more receptive to other people being funny too? If I'm going to laugh out loud, though - in other words, show the world I found something funny - it has to be properly good stuff.

I have no problem laughing at things on TV or the cinema, as I forget about my surroundings. I laugh less often in company as I feel more 'on show' and self-conscious. I tend to laugh out loud more at things I shouldn't, that suddenly strike me as funny and so catch me unawares. Unfortunately, I have no problem guffawing then!

As for the humour we're meant to like, painted with the broad brush strokes, I like that as much as more sensitive humour. I can laugh at Laurel and Hardy, cartoons, kids' movies (love those). I also laugh at the more off-beat humour in programmes like Fringe.

Yes, readers, **I love finding things funny**. It's a release, it lifts you up, frees you for a moment. It makes you feel good and is a great way to connect with other people. You may not know what to say to them but if you can find the same thing funny or can make them laugh, you're half way to being friends.

In my darkest times, I made a concerted effort to bring light into the darkness, to keep it at bay, prod it, spike it, pierce it until the sun shone through. Have at you, darkness, you can't beat me! Not today, not while I have this laughter in my heart!

I want to grow into my different stages of life still laughing, still smiling at the pleasures of a small, instant, funny-goose. I want to have laughter lines and for people to see my teeth when I find something funny. I want to make it funny for them too, as I know everyone has those dark parts of the day.

Let us not need caffeine to buzz through the day. Let's be silly, subtle or sensitive in our laughter. Just give in to it and see things in a different way.

Lastly, I'm not saying all aspies have a sense of humour. I've discovered, bizarrely, that some people don't like funnies. Some of those people may be aspies. I've also discovered some people don't watch Fringe either. The world is a strange place.

What I would say is, don't assume aspies can't see the humour-geese. Those geese get everywhere and are often only seen by the person right next to them. For all you know, that stony-faced woman in the queue behind you is looking blank because she's enjoying some private joke, re-visiting a funny scene or waiting to share a goose with someone else.

Don't judge a joke by its cover, readers. And don't forget to poke your pointy stick at the darkness, for you and other people.

It's an aspie on the phone...

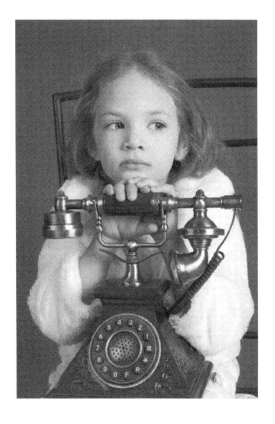

'Madam, your deadline was the 5th of this month...'

A pause so that I can insert the stupendously important reason why I didn't send my forms back in time. The call centre person is waiting, his tone has been efficient and officious since I was put through and he obviously expects a really good answer for my complete lack of organisation. What can I say?

I flash through the options in that super-quick way you develop after so very many years of having to think of on-the-spot excuses. Oh well, none of them will sound good.

I reply with a simple, 'Yes,' agreeing with him. I know the deadline was the 5th.

There is another pause. Call centre people aren't used to this. They can deal with lateness but only if you offer reasons and they are trained to filter the excuses from the reasons too. It's something like quality control but without much quality by the end.

There is a slight sigh, then I'm told, 'The deadline has passed so you will need to re-submit the form and the date will be from when we receive it.'

I sigh too, but hide it - sighing from the customer implies sorrowful acceptance of my fate or worse, criticism of the call centre. When you miss as many deadlines as I do, you learn to make the call centre person your ally, if possible.

'I know, I realise that,' I say sadly, falling back on my stalwart approach of sounding sad and as if I have a very good but hidden reason for being foolish, one I am unable to share with them. This sad air of mystery has dragged me out of many troublesome holes.

There is another pause and I hear clicking from his end as he types something onto my file.

'Madam, if you can return the form within four days, we should be able to keep the break to a week at most. Can you return it within that time?'

'Yes, thank you!' I sigh audibly this time, with glad relief. 'I will definitely get it back to you in four days!'

I now sound absurdly grateful, as if I am on the verge of being offered his daughter's kidney. I let my voice waver a little, to show I am moved by the kindness and his tone changes to one of concern as well as helpfulness. He is my ally now.

The rest of the call is spent in the usual organising noises, slotted in to make sure your telephonic visit is as turgid as possible. I ring off, finally, eventually, totally free of the call and make myself find the stupid form and fill in the stupid boxes and replace the stupid envelope I lost, which was the reason I dilly-dallied and never sent it back on time. There, it goes in my bag so he can receive it in four days and mitigate my latest disaster.

Sometimes, though, I think how easy it would be if, in the pause they leave for my reason, I could slot in, 'I am an Aspie, I do these things.' Life is never that simple though and if I was to use my Aspergers as a reason for missing a deadline, then it would become awkward. I would have to explain myself, expose a private part of my life and then hear the other person's tone of voice change as they decide how to handle this strange and rather alarming piece of information.

I always end up leaving it just so, letting them think I am a flake instead, a woman with problems, a sad-voiced individual who somehow manages to stretch the deadline and enact that little-used policy they have in their power.

Readers, if only people in my real life were as easily handled then things would be much simpler. How ironic that I can use this people-reading skill so adeptly in moments of call centre crisis but not when my nearest and dearest are bearing down on me with my latest sin.

That's how it goes, I suppose. If my super power must be Deadline Stretching, then I guess I can still make the world a better place, one missed form at a time.

Phone vs People

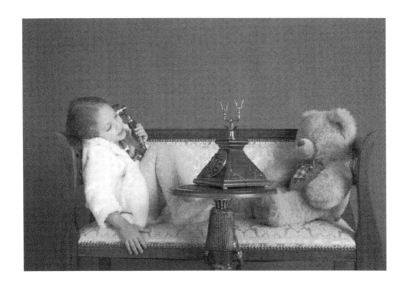

Before I say anything more, I must point out that I do not like talking to people on the phone. I don't even like talking to computers on the phone, or being passed to my mother's cat so I can hear it purr. Phones are Not Good, an intrusion into my safe place, an invention designed to wheedle us out into the open without ever having to leave our dens. So, it was with some surprise when I discovered I could 'do' phones.

I always detested using them in my many jobs and did avoid using my home phone too. Any calls I made were kept short and simple, often with much face-pulling at my end as I worked out where the conversation was going. Then I started doing private tuition and I turned a corner.

When people call me to tutor their children, they need to know what kind of a person I am. As well as the usual questions, our chat helps them to find out if they can connect with me, enabling them to suss out my personality and test that feeling you have when you decide whether or not you might like someone.

I have always been polite and friendly with them but at first I concentrated on seeming professional. I didn't want them to think I was a charlatan and I focused on talking about the work I would do to help their child overcome problems.

Then I had a call from someone who I just couldn't seem to focus on in that way. It was the mother of a new student and she was just terrible at this phone business. She wanted what was best for her child and asked a couple of questions but then kept faltering off and leaving awkward silences. This meant I had to go on a friendly offensive to find out what she wanted to know.

We were on the phone quite a long time and I managed to filter down to what she needed and what she wanted to know about me before I turned up for the first lesson. She told me a few times she didn't like talking on the phone but she was forced to sometimes (so I knew her awkwardness wasn't personal to me).

It was a breakthrough for me as I realised that I was not the only one who hated the dreaded phone and also I found I could take charge of a conversation, guiding it and the other person to the right place by the end. Ta-da!

From then on I made sure to inject more of my own personality into the calls, as well as drawing out the personality of the potential client. I found out that I could do this by listening intently to *how* they said things, rather than *what* they said. It was like a kind of empathic exploration, which is ironic considering all the times my lack of empathy has let me down in my real-life conversations.

The phone, it seemed, was a conduit. The conversations I found so very difficult face-to-face became entirely possible when everything was channelled through my ears.

Call centre experiences became much easier as I treated the other person like one of my clients, listening and reacting to them to see what I should say next. I have diffused quite a few potential problems in my life using this method and even won the help of some supremely unhelpful call centre employees.

Over time I learned to project the most useful part of my personality, such as in the previous chapter when I became sad and helpless. I could judge what was most beneficial to the conversation – with most problems it is best to be genuinely in need, as most people do step out to help you. But quite often I have to bolster my usual mild responses and make myself formidable, unstoppable, efficient, so that the call centre person will take notice of me.

There is always an emotional drain after these calls – they are not simply made and then forgotten. Much as I come across like a normal person on the phone, once I have replaced the receiver I am relieved and need to settle back into my safe place. Being the right kind of person is exhausting.

Personal calls

I must add that this doesn't work so well in personally difficult conversations; it seems the emotional aspect sabotages my reactions. Although I can work out what the other person is wanting to say, my own responses revert to stumbling gaffes and terrorised silences. It is like I become the shy, anxious child again, allowing the other person to lead because I have no idea where we are going.

Thanks to this emotional stutter, I have had many calls where the other person gets their own way, or has free rein to be as obnoxious as they like without any real resistance from me. I know when it is happening that I should be speaking up but there is a barrier, an unseen force set carefully between me and my honesty.

And readers, if I could speak in these conversations I would do one of two things: I would either state the facts and not deviate, which doesn't bode well for an emotional conversation anyway, or I would simply say, 'You are bullying me, I don't want to talk to you.' There again, we have a failed conversation.

What happens is that I withdraw, which leaves the other person able to say whatever they like. I allow them to spew emotions down the phone, let them carry on like babies babbling at the rattle, just because I am not *here*, not connected to this place. The phone becomes what it always was, a hard, unyielding object placed in my home to enable invaders to access my safe space.

Leave a message

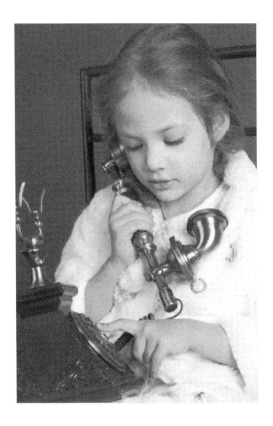

Many times I ignore the phone, even when I know who calls (sometimes especially when I know who calls). I like people to leave a message, let me know what they want so I can rush to the virtual dressing-up box and pull out the right thing to wear.

If I just pick up the phone and listen, then I might grab the wrong accessory and be over-dressed, ready to go to the ball when my caller wants to talk about the price of eggs. If I hesitate, letting them talk while my hand wavers over the dressing-up box, then I am in danger of choosing nothing at all and having one of those conversations where I come across as monotone and detached.

It is very tempting, when answering the phone and having to react immediately, to switch off as much as possible. There is no real escape, not with the phone lodged in your hand. You could walk off and leave it sitting there with the tinny little voice seeping out. Or you could put your hand over the receiver and pretend you never picked it up.

Instead, when there is no way out and I am unable to formulate the correct reaction, I either take a while to warm up or I go bland and grey. Warming up is kind of okay, if you have enough time to redeem the conversation. Usually people remember how you were at the end of the call so if you manage to enliven your reactions and become part of the conversation, people will remember you this way.

If you find it almost impossible to respond and simply interact as little as possible, then you are in danger of entering the territory of the slow voice, the grey tone, the overcast skies of nothing much at all. The conversation is irrelevant; you are detached from it, present only because you picked up the phone. You are not yourself and the other person is not real either.

They talk and their words tumble out of the phone, falling silently around you as you wait for them to finish. The letters pile up, a messy heap that you might deal with later. The conversation carries on only as long as the other person can keep it going. If they are intent on giving you information or they are worked up about their subject, then it takes longer for them to realise how detached you are. If they called specifically to get a reaction from you, they will notice almost straight away that you are not connecting with them.

Sometimes it is very hard to work up a reaction, even if you know it is expected. There are times when it wouldn't matter who called you and what they called about, you would still feel disconnected and grey. You are capable of listening to what they tell you and even of taking it in - where you fail is in reacting appropriately.

This is not even honesty, readers; this is not boredom or displeasure. It is a grey feeling which settles like dank, heavy snow and stops you from being able to become part of the conversation. It can happen face to face too but I find it much more common on the phone.

And then we are uncaring again and feelings are hurt. We are supposed to care, supposed to be friends. They are there for us and where are we? At the other end of a phone, no less, with the type of voice that says even the end of the world is preferable to this call.

Leave a message, please. Leave it and be detailed. Do not ask me to call you back without any clues as to why you called. If I wanted surprises I would not be this person. If I wanted to be caught off-guard then I would not use my answer-phone.

177

Tell me why you called, tell me what you want, tell me all about it and be as excitable as you like. By the time I call you back I will have rearranged my reaction and will project more of what you hoped for when you first called. I will have hidden the grey monotone away and will be wary of it, watching for it emerging before the end of the call.

Leave me a message and I will do my best to answer your call with the personality you expect. Don't take it to heart, you are still special. But leave a message and let me relax, knowing what you want before I have to speak to you about it. Let me be prepared, that is all. It's a small thing and it makes my colours brighter.

The sound of a thousand voices
quietened by a single click

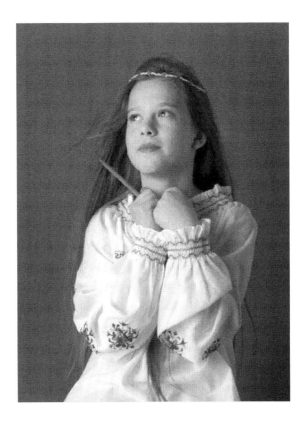

I want to talk about shutting down, turning off, zoning out, being absent...all things aspies know about (and love, by the way, don't believe it if they say they don't).

Every aspie is able to zone out, often so completely and utterly you think, where did that aspie of mine go? Didn't I leave one here a minute ago? Am I alone? Oh no, wait, that lump leaning lovingly against the computer screen, that's where I left it. This thought or feeling can cross your mind even when the great lump of aspie is stood in front of you, blocking out the light, supposedly listening to the very important thing you have to tell them.

I'm talking about a **total disconnect**, the sort of shut down, however short, that means all-out war could descend on your house and you'd have to sling your beloved over your shoulder to get them out because it would be quicker than gaining their attention and keeping their attention while escaping from the war-zone.

I don't experience this shutdown as often as I used to. Being a busy mother, daughter, pet-keeper and self-employed do-er, I have to be partially plugged in for most of the time. And, let's face it, if I did zone out, I wouldn't know, would I? But I can still zone out enough, for different reasons, to make life exciting.

For now, though, I want to travel back in time, to show how all-encompassing this shutdown can be. Let me be clear - I was probably an odd child but I still managed school (by the skin of my teeth), I made friends (the sort who like odd friends) and I would be classed now as high-functioning and gifted. So, I was made for surviving but not always for life as we know it.

One day, I went to play with my friend after school. For a change we went to her grandparents' house in a local village. This was the kind of village where the mist descends when everywhere else is in sunshine and where you most certainly have to be local to be accepted. My friend counted as local; I did not.

We met up with some children she knew in the school yard. The girls were quite friendly and we were having a nice time. Then a boy came who they all knew and didn't like. They looked at me, worried, then back at him. He liked to cause trouble you see.

Now, to be honest, by the time he showed up, I had already been losing interest in what was going on. When he arrived, the conversation changed. I lost the final bit of interest and away I went. I have no idea where. As I was about 9 it probably involved ponies or Doctor Who. Wherever it was, I was happy and stayed there for some time. I was engrossed, the inner world had me good and proper and I had no idea where I was or who I was with.

For some reason, I drifted back to the mortal plane and found myself in the centre of a shocked silence. The boy was looking triumphantly at me, my friend looked like she was waiting for me to cry and her two friends were horrified. These were tough cookies so I knew something must be up for them to be so affected.

I looked around at them, taking in the strained faces and the gleeful bully-boy.

'What?' I asked, mystified. The last time I checked in, no one was even talking to me.

'Are you okay?' One of the tough cookie girls asked, a hand on my arm and her face sympathetic.

'Yes...' I answered, giving her a little smile.

'She's hiding it well, she must be really upset,' someone else said.

'Upset about what?' I was starting to worry; had something happened?

It turns out the nasty boy had said something so bad they chased him off and escorted me back to my friend's grandparents' house, all the while praising me for being so brave and saying I didn't have to pretend, that it was okay to be upset.

When I was finally alone with my friend, I managed to convince her that I hadn't heard any of it and was completely innocent. But I was so curious! What a reaction! What had I missed?

She believed me when I told her I didn't know and, being the most down-to-earth friend I've ever had, she wouldn't tell me. No amount of persuasion would bring it out. She said if I didn't know then there was no need to tell me, I would only get upset.

To this day, I have no idea what was said, I just know that being an aspie who was bored at the time, with an inner-life strong enough to draw me in and hold me close, I was saved from something that would probably have been bad enough to haunt me to this day. The atmosphere was so strong when I came back; the faces are what I remember, even though I couldn't tell you who the girls were. It was a dreadful thing and I was saved from it.

Other things have happened since, other pieces of life's cruelty have not been swept away by my ability to leave and return. Those cruelties have stayed with me and cut deeply for a very long time afterwards. I often think how grateful I am that I was spared that one, the words of a bully which would have cut me deep enough to bring forward the sympathy of strong, tough girls and to make my faithful friend keep it to herself for as long as I knew her.

Dear readers, I offer no solutions for the closing off from the 'real' world. I accept this retreat as a blessed thing. It is truly wonderful to be able to escape such a complex, confusing, noisy and intimidating place as the world we aspies inhabit every day. Even a partial shutdown is enough to carry you through and make life bearable again.

I realise how it can seem from the outside. You know the ears work, the tongue works, the body works when it chooses to move; and yet it does not speak, will not listen, makes no sign it heard you. I can imagine you feel alone and left out and probably hurt. I'm so sorry for it, we don't mean to hurt you.

Please take comfort from the fact that if we *did* succeed and could stay in this world, with you, on a permanent basis, we would not be the same beloved. We would be sadder and more stressed, the world would be an even harsher place and, with time, you would seem part of that harshness for making us be there always.

It's okay, we're still here. We can be frustrating when you need us to be present but don't worry. What you lose in those moments is regained in the peace we feel while we're away. And it's that peace which gives us the strength to be more fully ourselves when we are here.

Seeing the whole person

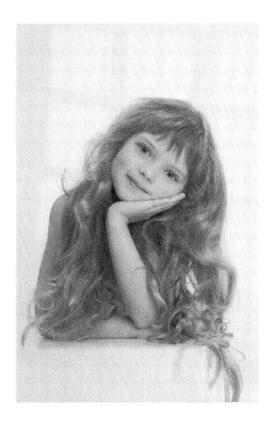

They say if you want to see a room as it really is, mess and all, you should take a picture and look at that. They say that it's too easy to miss the obvious when you see it all the time and you need to look at it a different way to see it clearly.

So, your living room, which you just cleaned today, is transformed in a photograph. You suddenly see the biscuit wrappers on the sofa, the bundle of dog hair on the corner of the rug, the peeling paint on the radiator and the place where the cat scratched at the door frame when he was little.

All these things are meant to be invisible to those of us who are permanently distracted. We see what we think there is to be seen and anything else is left to be noticed by visitors.

I was thinking the same approach might be useful for Life. Imagine if you could hold a cosmic camera and take a picture of your life, as it really is? Putting aside the fact we humans are only meant to know so much and would probably be driven insane by the unadulterated truth, what would we see that is not obvious now?

Would we suddenly see all those things other people have been telling us about for years? Would I understand, finally, what my mother means by me not getting round to things? Would the confusion at my inability to cope evaporate if I could know the truth of my life?

In fact, would my life become more understandable to me or other people?

It's nice to think that the cosmic camera could show my life to others in a way that might help them understand the aspie point of view, as well as the whole gamut of difficulties and impossibilities that follow us around like angry chickens.

I'd like to think that this truth-inducing picture would be there as proof that I have not slacked off, I am not to blame for everything that went wrong, that I really did do my best here, and here, and that little bit there too.

It's a cosy image, this idea that you could show others how it really is, without the need for explanations or arguments. Just push a well-thumbed photograph into their hand and wait for their face to change as they see what it was like.

I guess this is the dream of perfect understanding from other people. Aspies want to feel justified in not being able to cope, seeming to goof off or shuffle into the undergrowth at the first sign of trouble. We want others to see it as we do and not judge us so harshly.

However, I have a feeling that any such picture, taken by the cosmic camera, would be for our eyes only. Madness lies in complete understanding, but by understanding ourselves completely, we could reach perfect sanity in our own tiny space in the universe.

We couldn't show the picture to anyone else as they'd only see an underwhelming portrait of us, smiling manically at the camera. They wouldn't see what we did, they wouldn't understand our need to have their ultimate approval.

With the picture in our hand, though, we might be strong at last. We could cast off the uncertainty and leave behind the quivers as we faced what and who we are without the need to explain ourselves. We would be able, after so long, to have that silent moment where everything falls into place.

What might happen afterwards would be revolutionary. Imagine yourself unshackled at last, armed with self-understanding and the knowledge you needed to tackle life without losing sight of who you really are. The bliss of such an existence!

And yet, readers, this is what we strive for every day. All the little sufferings I know you go through, all the times you clasp your hands together in anxiety, wishing there was someone to unclasp them and hold them instead. All of those times when you wish it would stop and you could re-start, afresh, a new person, leaving behind the sharp stings of being.

All of these things, painful, annoying, upsetting, confusing, they are part of the cosmic photograph we have been given. We can never take the picture ourselves but we are allowed to look at it. The trouble is, we can never look at it all at once so we are forced, step by step, day by day, to look at one piece at a time.

Eventually, after a lot of steps and time taken to study what we can see, we can put together a mental image of the whole photograph. It is possible to finally see yourself as complete, without needing the explanations, without feeling the pain of who you are.

It is true that it takes some time to reach this stage and, just to keep life interesting, that photograph never stays exactly the same. Be comforted and know that it does happen. If you strive for understanding and a clear, honest, loving vision of yourself, you will see who you are and why.

And readers, it will be a wonderful picture.

6: Learning to Communicate

I cannot stress this enough: aspies learn from what they observe around them and this education continues right through life. There is no cut-off point where we think, 'There, now I am fully formed'. Aspies understand they will always have something new to learn and never more so than when it comes to understanding other people. This book may be called How to Talk to Your Aspie, but it is written after many years where I have had to learn how to talk to other people and understand what they were saying back.

In the short term, aspies learn how a person behaves and what they are likely to say. They can be more or less confident that good old Bruce won't throw a temper tantrum if he doesn't get his magazine on time or that Gloria should not be kept waiting if she invited you over for coffee. Aspies see the bigger, broader strokes of Bruce being patient and Gloria being impatient. They also see how Bruce's eyes crinkle when he explains what you did wrong or that Gloria's eyes blaze with barely-disguised fury if you clinked her good china cup against the side of the coffee pot.

Aspies learn all the time and re-evaluate what they see of the world as they go. They also learn from a young age that being wrong comes naturally, that the world is difficult to understand and that other people can be reliably unpredictable. That is not to say that all people are unpredictable;

rather that to aspies they seem unpredictable because their behaviours seem hard to understand.

Coping mechanisms are adopted to protect against this unpredictability and so if Bruce was to suddenly snap and lose his temper, a part of the aspie would not be surprised, even though the behaviour would be shocking. We come to expect the unexpected, being aware of only part of the picture and not seeing the whole of people at first glance.

If you only see part of the picture then at some stage the big reveal may be a nasty (or nice) surprise. Until we have that big reveal, we can only work with the information we have gathered so far. And if we have been told growing up that we should not react in a particular way to this big reveal, then we will try to modify our behaviour accordingly.

In other words, we have learned that it is unacceptable to panic or have a tantrum when people seem inexplicable because it is unreasonable to behave in this way. We should understand people if we have known them for long enough; everyone else can understand them.

This section deals with how we react and how much of it is learned behaviour, actually at odds with our own natural personality. Not being yourself is something that is forced upon many aspies and is another source of stress. Even when you are with people who want you to be wholly yourself, it is second nature to behave in the way you found worked best when you were growing up.

No matter whether we react or over-react, aspies have to confront a world with particular expectations and then we also have to communicate with that world. Barriers upon barriers come between us and somewhere along the line we open our mouths and say what we feel is necessary. We mimic self-expression because real expression has had dire consequences in the past. And then we walk away, confused.

The world is my family, because I know nothing else.

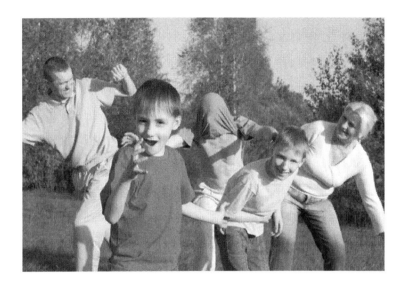

Treat others as you want to be treated, remember? Haven't we all had this explained to us at some stage, by well-meaning souls or angry best beloveds when they found out we told work they'd had a duvet day. But what about treating others as *they* expect to be treated?

In the aspie world, we learn by example, often because our own experience and knowledge seems at odds with what other people know. If we see our powerful parents doing something a certain way, then that becomes the right way to do it. This is true of all children, but let me explain why it becomes more true of the aspie.

Over time, other children learn by their own experiences. Aspies aren't immune to this. We also learn some of the many and complex methods of living in the modern world. Then we come up against a barrier. It's an invisible one, created gently by our younger years when so many 'rules' were set in place.

Over time, other children grow and understand that life isn't always what you expect or were even led to believe. The nursery teacher who said we should all be friends was right but she was wrong when she said we *could* all be friends.

The parent who says we should be considerate at the dinner table was right but when they said this is how all people behaved, they were wrong. Growing up, a parent who says this is what all people do, so you must do it, is instilling a lesson they think will help their little one. They don't often do it for spite, you know? Yet later, when we realise some people trough like pigs at the dinner table, the aspie knows this is wrong, knows it is at odds with what they were taught but fails to understand that other people, the piggy-troughers, will see it as wholly acceptable.

It is this ability to see the other point of view where we fall down. While we were young and spongey, our parents helped us to see life their way and learn from them. What we learned above all else was that our parents knew everything. Fast forward to an aspie adult and there is still a child in there, believing the parental world view.

If this world view stops you from jumping queues or eating off the floor, it's a good thing. The problem comes when you don't know why other people do these things and why, when you put them straight, they don't appreciate your help.

I believe that aspies expect the whole world to be like their family. The way they learned to live from an early age is how the world should be. We do understand that other people get it wrong but we don't quite figure out why they don't want to have it put right.

This blinkered view is over and above any personality traits of the aspie themselves. They may be the most laid back, non-OCD aspie there is, willing to love the world and greet them as friends, but within lies the child who feels, even if they don't believe, that the way their parents did it is the proper way to live.

And there is the crux of the matter, where logic cannot shine. While aspies are good at feeling things, they are often pretty bad at explaining or dissecting those feelings. If we feel a certain way, we know it's a truth because it's right there, in the middle of the chest, making you fill with emotion that doesn't leave room for any argument. A good person might come to you and explain why you feel this way and why it isn't necessarily the truth, but will you listen? Even if you try?

Our upbringing, with the all-knowing family members, never stops affecting the way we see the world. Even if you know your family was wrong or what they did was mad, it still feels right to do the same because it's what you know.

Even if there is a moment, every day, where you have to stand and give yourself a talking to so you can behave how you want and not how you were taught, you will always be followed around by what you once knew to be the ultimate truth.

The world is my family, because I know nothing else. My family showed me how to live when I knew nothing. It made me understand what seemed incomprehensible. It loved me when no one else cared. And now, as an aspie adult, I'm supposed to shuck off that knowledge and teaching and take on a new one, so that I can work better in the world and feel better too?

Yes, that is what we have to do. Every adult aspie has a responsibility to their inner child to keep on growing and learn new truths, even if those truths have to squeeze in next to the old ones. Sometimes, inner compromise and balance is the greatest gift we can give ourselves as adults.

Don't train your aspie!

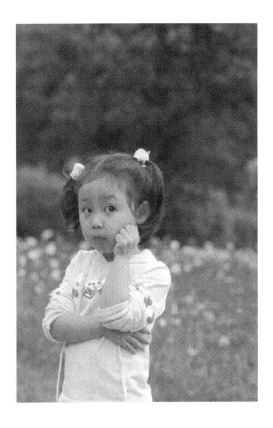

You know how they say, if you hear something often enough, you start to believe it? I was torturing myself with some past *stuff* last night, caught up in replay mode, where you know you've heard it a thousand times before, a bit like granny's stories of when she told Mrs so-and-so just what she thought of her, but can you stop it? Of course not.

It's not just at night. Through the day, in normal life, the replay starts and you hear the old voices, the familiar phrases. Most of them tell a 'truth' about you, something you learned growing up or which formed part of a significant relationship.

One of my truths was always that I was not practical, followed by the well-worn and amusing diatribe on how the practical gene skipped a generation, how my children would probably get it instead. And then the sideways jump to how it didn't skip past my cousins though - at which point I'd be likened to my great-grandmother, who preferred her gardening to keeping the house clean and tidy. She died a heroine so I never minded that too much.

Except, when I've become more assertive with age (and it took a loooong time), I discovered that while every nail I knocked in was likely to bounce back out, I was very good at looking at the bigger picture and showing other people where to put the nails.

This often meant I was seen as being critical too, even though my reasoning usually solved some difficult problem that the practical people had spent an hour scratching their heads about. It was obvious to me but being so resolutely *not* practical, I stayed away until the sound of cursing and nails being removed was too much to bear.

As a non-practical person, I have also been pushed away from sites of busy-ness and doing, as if my very presence would hold up the fine industry of real people, the ones who *can* knock in a nail. 'Here, get out of the way!' was the usual phrase, or 'Can you not do anything but stand there and look?'

If you get used to being sent off or made to take part (rather than stand and look), you start removing yourself from the situation. You grow accustomed to sitting in another room and listening to the sound of those hammers working away with the kind of industry that built empires (and you know how they usually turn out).

You become adept at reading through the disturbance, or pushing refreshments through the gap in the door so you won't be drawn in to helping or told off for being there at the wrong moment. And, you really, really get used to admiring other people's shoddy handiwork because you know you couldn't have done it half as well yourself.

In other words, you train yourself to step back and only take part when it's all over, by which time you have no choice but to say it looks good. You have no room for manoeuvre once you have vacated the situation.

If you have the courage to stay and help in your own way, not by wielding the hammer but by looking at things from your unique perspective, then you have a far greater chance of helping out. You can often make things better than by leaving the room. However - and this is a big however - this only works if the nail-hitters will allow you to help in your *own way*.

If they insist on doing it their way, on your space in the plan being dictated by how they see the world, then you will do little to help and might make things worse. Blaming you for your part in this compounds your feelings of helplessness and detachment, making it less likely you will be involved the next time.

So, taking part in situations you have been trained to avoid does take courage and not just on your part. Other people need to put down the hammer occasionally and consider there may be a better way to make the world than by fixing one plank at a time. They also need to be brave enough to look at their aspie and say, 'What do you think? Is there anything else I can do?'

And then, they have to listen to the answer too.

First thoughts, second thoughts, third thoughts...

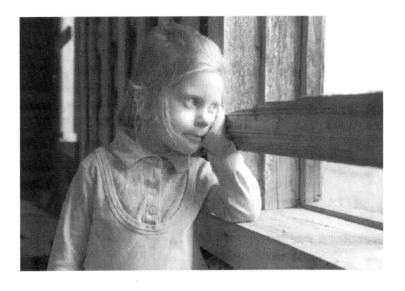

First thoughts, second thoughts, third thoughts. How many times can one person come along the same road and see the same landmarks and try to look at them in a new way? Lots of times, if you want to know the truth.

To an extent, everyone second guesses themselves; it's a part of life and makes humanity an occasional great thinker. The main reasoning behind re-thinking is to explore a subject, to see it from all possible angles and ultimately to make a judgement about it.

Less satisfactory is that excessive over- thinking leads to an inability to make decisions or to re-visiting past events as if you could have done something differently. You know you can't go back and change things, yet you see what might have been, almost as if it *can* be changed.

This way of obsessing over subjects and events is closely linked with self-esteem and self-doubt, sometimes forming a part of the internal aspie processes to such an extent that decisions can rarely be made without being pored over first.

If you are already thinking through how to do things on a daily basis, even with situations that are familiar to you, it's not surprising that you plod repeatedly through other events and experiences when they don't occur all the time.

Aspies have a need to make things familiar, even if they've never done them before or have no real way of knowing how things will turn out.

Similar to a wedding rehearsal, the aspie plots out the variables of a future-something to see if they can make it a little more routine, with the expected outcomes branched out neatly on a mental diagram. A map for life, perhaps?

If the event has already happened and something went wrong, or feels wrong and makes the aspie uneasy, it will be re-played on the internal super-computer. This can be the case even if we know exactly what went wrong and don't doubt the outcome. If the event has been in any way disturbing, it will be re-visited.

This isn't the same as lying in your bed, flicking through regrets. It can be applied to anything, just so that life makes a little more sense. It's a way of bringing meaning out of potential chaos.

If the event went the right way but was dramatic enough to impact on the aspie psyche, then it will be thought through again, just to examine it, to turn it over and see if there's anything that went unnoticed the first time.

This is a way to understand life, other people, our reactions to them. We are always searching for hidden meaning; we assume there *is* hidden meaning, even in everyday happenings, because so much of meaning is already hidden from us.

I think this need to re-think and re-visit is fundamental to an aspie's sense of security too. There's the childish belief, not often expressed, that if you can think about and visualise something enough, it will lose its power over you and you will be in control.

Rather like when children imagine what they would do in a dangerous situation - they have their actions planned out and are the champion of the story. It's the children who don't have an exit strategy you have to worry about, as it's a sign they feel powerless. As children, we are already powerless, so this planning ahead and imagining is a way of coping with that, of denying it and by denying it, making it not true.

As an adult aspie, we know that by thinking things through, however many times, we can't make them true or untrue. If they have already happened, it's too late anyway. If they are still to come, we have enough life experience to realise these things have a will of their own and are not often in our control.

And yet still we think, and consider, and wonder, and make decisions based on these internal musings which sometimes have little connection with the reality of the situation. Whole life decisions can be based on what an aspie imagines will happen and whether that inner visualisation has enough power to seem true.

I guess you might say that Aspergers comes with its own, in-built quantum generator. We don't manufacture whole universes but we do create endless possible scenarios of this one, so that we can filter through them and see what the future might hold. Or see what might have been if we had acted differently in our past.

It's very dangerous territory, to picture a potential future borne from an undone past. The fictional future was never meant to be and yet it holds an allure for the aspie in trouble, or denial, as it whispers to you, *'this might have been your life, this could have been yours.'*

It can be a useful tool to watch and listen to these numerous thoughts on how things might be, or have been. Acting with self-knowledge and kindness, we can use these imaginary lifelines to learn new things about ourselves and what we really want from the world.

Look out for the complete re-write, though. That's the one you need to avoid. It can have you living a perfect life, with great hair and everything just so, if only you had done this instead of that. Life doesn't work that way, for anyone.

No matter what your logic tells you, life cannot be held up to the sun and peered at without squinting. If you could see everything clearly, without the squint, you would not be able to understand the vast possibilities. What would be the point of living if you knew everything and never made mistakes? What would there be left to learn?

Have the first thoughts, second thoughts, third thoughts. Be a little wary by the time you reach the fourth and fifth. Keep an eye on yourself beyond that. Use the inner visualisation to help yourself, not to fill out the jowls of winky old regret.

Become wiser, readers, even if your wisdom only helps you understand yourself. And if you do stray into those other universes, be kind to yourself when you get there.

It's rude to stare...

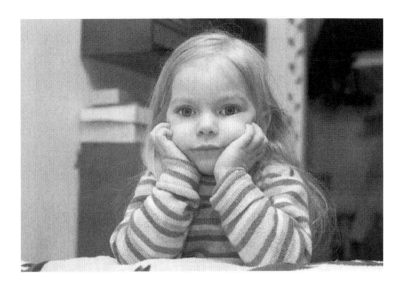

I had lunch with my mother and step-sister yesterday. I always have mixed feelings before I go as I know I'll end up on the outside looking in, with that sensation of being in the wrong place, as if I was meant to end up somewhere else and forgot along the way.

It's like that when we're all together. I am there, on one side, and somehow my mother and step-sister are on the other. Their conversations swirl and eddy and I sit, wondering if I should participate or just let them get on with it (as usual).

It's strange how this feeling of isolation can happen so frequently when you're with your nearest and dearest, surrounded by people who would literally drop everything to rush to your side if you needed them. It's kind of like a stupid joke where the reality is they are a faithful, loyal family but the everyday logic tells you they are also separate.

I listened to the conversation, waiting for cues to join in and trying to keep my face animated for when their gazes scanned across the table to include me. This didn't last long as I happened to notice a strange shade in my step-sister's hair colour and spent most of my time trying to figure out if it was a bad dye job or she had started to go grey.

My eye could not leave that patch of colour alone. Every chance I got I was staring at it, then tracing it back to her parting to see if it joined up with any grey there. And, like the eye of Sauron, her gaze swivelled round just as I was getting a good look and I'd have to flinch away and find a fascinating point behind her. No wonder people avoid me.

I was then left with staring out of the window or at the old woman at the other table. Luckily, the old woman wasn't as observant as my step-sister but she wasn't as interesting either. Finally, as a desperate attempt to distract myself I offered my own piece of conversation.

You know, it wasn't a dull piece either. I regaled them with my Thursday schedule (it was more exciting than it sounds), adding the funny parts where I'll be falling asleep by the end of the day. I swear, readers, I swear I got the Polite Moment of Listening before they turned back to the turgid tale that had hogged lunch for most of our visit.

I sighed, had one last look at my step-sister's hair and then took out my phone and went onto Facebook. I know it's rude to go online while you're meant to be socialising and even worse to message people in the middle of lunch with your relatives. I considered this rudeness almost as briefly as they had given me the Polite Moment of Listening, then I put it aside.

There comes a time in life when you don't feel compelled to sit and suffer like before. The advent of mobile tech at least means we have an escape from these times and it really does save you from making your own entertainment by staring at things you shouldn't or derailing the conversation just because you're bored.

It wasn't long before I had to go and we all parted amicably. I came away with a smile on my face as I'd enjoyed those ten minutes on the phone. I'll go again, of course, but the next time I'll take the phone out sooner and save us all the embarrassment of me staring at the ceiling, right quick, as if I wasn't looking at anything else at all.

And I'm pretty certain it was a bad dye job after all.

The fear reaction

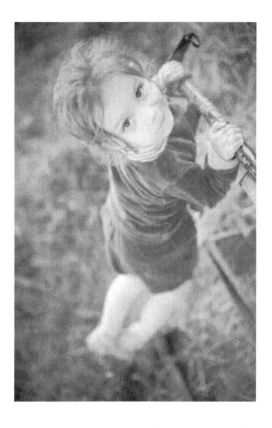

When I was little more than three years old, I almost died. It was a normal day which became suddenly dramatic. My mother and I were on holiday with an auntie and cousin. We went for a break in Morecambe, a seaside town in the North West of England.

We were walking along the pier and, as usual, I was running on ahead. We were heading for the end of the pier so I went at top speed to get there.

Halfway along there was a hole in the wood, at a point where there was a big drop and deep water underneath.

My mother has a distinct memory of one second I was running, then I was gone. I had run over the hole and just dropped.

Very luckily, my body thought for me and as I dropped I reached up and grabbed the railings near the top of the hole. When my mother and auntie hurtled along they found my little hands clasping the railings while the rest of me hung, waiting to be rescued.

I have no memory of this event, though I've heard it relayed many times. I don't think my mother ever quite got over the shock as it would have been the end if I had fallen. The water was deep and churned around the struts of the pier beneath and we used to go out of season, so it was cold too. I couldn't swim and probably wouldn't have been able to in the currents anyway. And the struts criss-crossed beneath the pier, so even worse, I might have been knocked unconscious on my way down.

Growing up and throughout my adult life, I've had a fear of falling. Ladders are a trial, I don't mind stairs but am afraid of walking or driving next to steep drops. Even the curly roads up through multi-storey car parks bring me out in a sweat.

In the ice and snow, I either clothe my feet in over-the-top snow shoes or make little old lady steps wherever I go as I have a deep fear of falling over, even from my small height.

So, although I don't remember it, thanks to the replays from my mother and, quite possibly, a subconscious memory of the event, I hold within me a fear of falling and of deep water.

With therapy, I guess I might get past these but I don't think staying away from heights or deep water is necessarily a bad thing. What has been difficult is the unexplained fears which arise because of it. Not unexplained exactly, as I know where they come from, but when you are trying to climb a ladder to put up Christmas decorations, or to trim the hedge, people do tend to think you're being very silly if you start to wobble and need to cling on, like a cat up a tall tree.

Even with the justification of my smaller self almost dying, people think you should get over it. After all, it's not as if you remember it properly and no harm was done, right?

I let them think what they like, readers, as I'm not for budging on this one. Why should I bend to peer pressure and place myself in a situation where I know I'll lose sight of reason and give in to fear, so putting myself in danger?

This is how it can be with Aspergers in life too - and it isn't as tenuous a connection as it seems.

With Aspergers we learn what is scary at an early age and all our fears are reinforced as we grow. With me, I learned to fear social situations as other

215

people do what they like and I'm stuck in the middle of the maelstrom with no way out.

This feeling of no control is exacerbated by the rules of acceptable behaviour: if you go somewhere to be social, you don't just throw your drink in the bin and leave. You don't lose your temper through sensory overload and yell (then leave). You don't hide in the toilets so long that people think you *have* left. You don't hide behind your best beloved or nearest ample relative and hope no one notices you until it's time to leave.

Basically, it's not acceptable to leave, so you end up staying.

This is facing the fear, is it not? Well, no. This is the equivalent of me climbing the ladder to trim the hedge. I set up the ladder so it won't move, I look at it and mentally shake my fist at it. I know it's not very high and I can trim that hedge. It won't take long and I'll be proud of myself when it's over.

Except that even climbing the steps makes the ladder vibrate and I am reminded that it is a movable object, a thing designed to be folded up and put away. I am not on solid ground and even though I've done all I can to make it safe, I still feel the slight movement and I know I have to be careful.

All the way up (and all the way into the social situation), I get on with what I have to do. Soon after, I misjudge my balance and the ladder wobbles. I wobble with it, at a slightly different frequency and the ladder begins to shake.

In the social situation I have done something out of the ordinary and realised, either by the reactions of other people or by past experience, that I have stepped out of line. I panic a little and behave more unnaturally, then panic some more. It all starts to go wrong.

In my ladder scenario, this is where I stop *everything* and grip on, waiting for it to be still. Sometimes this works - mostly I feel the sweat pricking out on my brow and I close my eyes, hoping the panic will pass. Usually I climb down for a minute to recover before deciding if I'm going back up.

In the unfolding social drama, I also stop everything and become the odd person, motionless in the middle of the room. People might ask me if I'm feeling okay, assuming I'm ill, though they know by looking at me that ill isn't quite the right word. They want to help but are made uneasy by my behaviour and aren't sure what to do.

This is the place where I grip on and decide whether to carry on as if nothing has happened or climb back down and recover. When you are on your own, trimming the hedge, you have no one to please but yourself. In the social arena, you have to take account of other people.

The social equivalent of gripping the ladder while you regain your balance is the point when you will be approached and singled out for concern. Being able to leave and come back might help (though once free it's doubtful you would come back), but unlike your hedge, people do notice when you flee a room as if you're being chased.

Anything you do in a social situation feels as though you're making it worse and drawing more and more attention to yourself. This might not be true, you may not stand out as much as you think, but what is true is that it is a mirror of real-life, a solid fear of something which manifests as strange behaviour and reactions.

When you're reacting to learned fear, like the fear of falling or the fear of other people, you are reacting in a way that keeps you safe. If you fear falling, it makes sense to get down from the high place. If you worry about other people, leave the situation until you feel better. Both situations feel equally dangerous.

What helps is if you have someone to hold the ladder. I would prefer them to do it for me, to go up and trim the hedge while I am safely on the ground. For the ladder, this might work and is more acceptable. When it comes to social situations, you can't get other people to do it for you.

If you have to be there, let your supportive other be there too. Don't hide behind them (at least not physically, it makes people stare), but do let them hold things steady for you. Let them guide conversations or step in if you flounder. Let them be the kind hand on the ladder, stopping it from shaking even before it starts. Let them be there for you.

To this best beloved or good friend or sympathetic relative, I need to say one thing. Your kindness may be boundless and you may know your aspie as well as you know yourself, but one thing should be understood. Without wanting to sound ungrateful, if your aspie says 'Don't leave me alone' before you set off, then please, **Do not leave them alone**.

This is true of all situations where your aspie needs your support, social or otherwise. It is completely transferable. If they do not want to be left, do not leave them.

This is more important than I can tell you. The number of times I've gone somewhere with a supportive person, begging them not to leave me and they agree, genuinely and with sympathy. Then you get there and, sooner or later, they do leave you, for normal reasons. They go to get a drink or to the toilet or see someone they know and chat for a minute. *This is being left alone.*

To the non-aspie, being in the same room or briefly exiting for a natural reason is not the same as deserting their aspie. But it *is* the same thing. It's not that it only takes seconds for panic to set in ('But I was only gone a minute, what could go wrong?'). It's more that panic set in well before we got there and was only waiting for an excuse to burst out again. The sight of your safe person with their back turned to you, walking away, is all it takes. It's a terrifying image.

Ladders, people, everyday challenges; whatever nightmare sets off your adrenaline and makes you reach for safety, be aware it is a proper, understandable, sensible response. It may not feel like it and it may not be possible to explain that way, but it is.

For reasons known or unknown, this thing is a terror and must be stopped. It's a simple idea and reacting as you feel you should is the best response. You can worry about why you behaved that way later, when you're safe. For the moment, *be* safe, with or without the help of other people.

Yes, I am advocating flight instead of fight, readers. I know there are plenty of times when this isn't practical, but I also know we have no way of facing and subduing our fears if we are expected to do so in the middle of the fear itself. Our only hope of overcoming them is to be able to look back and see them from a safe distance. The next time you might be able to face them, or the time after that.

Finding out what scares you is the first step to overcoming it. Don't be bullied into being brave just because that's what everyone else does. They are not you and only you can say, without doubt, this is what scares me and I will not face it today.

The quiet voice

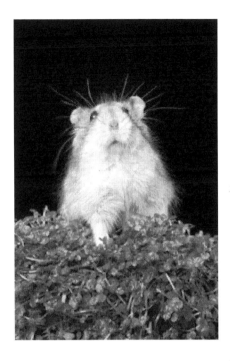

We've all been there, in the middle of a social occasion, surrounded by what might be called a friendly crowd. Someone makes a comment and, hey presto! it's something we know about. Bravery steps in, donning his floppy hat and swaggering briefly across our vision. Before we know it, we've broken our usual rules and spoken up - in a group!

Whatever we say, this time it's relevant, possibly witty, definitely in keeping with what went before. All yay, yay, yay!, especially compared to our usual experiences. And what happens? Absolutely nothing, that's what.

There's a short, blunt life lesson to be learned at many social gatherings: it doesn't matter what you say or how great a thing it is you have to share, you may be ignored as if you haven't spoken.

I'm calling this chapter 'The quiet voice' not because all aspies have quiet voices (though many do), but rather because our personalities and demeanour make our range shrink, pushing our influence to the outer edges of the group.

Unless we're in a group of close friends, it often happens that our voices are just not heard, or at least not *listened* to. Even if you're feeling super-confident about the conversation, which is unlikely, all the years of training yourself to stay out of the line of fire mean you have also trained yourself to be ignored.

We're not all little mousies, we don't have short trousers and soft, meek expressions. Some of us react to social situations by pulling faces, making awkward gestures or bizarre body language. This is the sort of thing usually guaranteed to get you attention. But I've often found that, despite my ability to stick out like a sore thumb when I least want it, at those times I would like to take part, I'm brushed aside as if I wasn't there,

I believe that the group, as a whole, is naturally geared towards the ones it sees as important. This is probably some kind of natural selection at work. After all, if you want the group to survive out on the plains, with the lions, you don't want some weirdy aspie who blinks too much in the sunshine and gets distracted by little bugs to be in charge when the roar suddenly comes from right behind you. I hold up my hands: it's fair to say that if aspies ruled the world, the human race would not be teeming everywhere like an upset ant-hill.

But you know, once you've chased the lions, eaten the antelope, made the babies and kept the camp fire going, you need the weirdy one to make life interesting. It isn't all about running, jumping, eating and mating. A lot of it is, I grant you that. What about the other bits though? The parts where you wonder about the stars or ask why the dandelion is yellow?

Who thought of all the questions? I'm not being funny here (all right, I am), but I don't think it was Mr Hunter, big enough to wrestle a lion and strong enough to drag it home. What do you think he thought about at night? Lions and women, in that order.

I'm also not saying all big thinkers were, or are, aspies. I will say that a lot of them probably were, though. To have the kind of sideways thinking that catapulted us towards the modern world, you would have to be wired up slightly differently from the norm.

And whose bright idea do you think it was to leave the forest and venture onto the plains in the first place? Do you think it was Mr Hunter, who was already hunting pretty well in the safety of the trees? Or was it an idea whispered in his ear by his quiet-voiced wife? Some little plan she had about spreading out, seeing what was beyond the forest, realising that lions were a necessary evil if they were to grow as people.

So many assumptions, I'll stick with what I know. When it comes to being heard, it can be very difficult as an aspie to be heard above the clamour of other people. They know without being told what to say first, to grab attention. They know the tricks of the vocal intonations aimed at cutting through the hubbub and taking the floor. They know where to stand or how to move so that their body language draws attention to them before they've even opened their mouth. They know the all-important clues that lead to other people seeing them, hearing them, understanding them.

Sometimes, if you're lucky, these clever, lucky people are also lovely people. I've watched as someone like this has taken centre stage, got everyone's attention, then told them they should listen to *me*. That's because you do come across people who have listened to the quiet voice and recognised it needs a little push in the right direction.

This is often how you find an aspie, awkward, quiet, desperately shy, being the friend of the over-confident, noisy loud-mouth.. People wonder what they see in each other. Do you want to know?

The loud-mouth is only loud because it suits them. It doesn't mean they're stupid or mean; they're just loud. They see in the aspie someone they can talk to, often without interruption. Not just a blank audience, mind you, the aspie is someone who listens carefully. While the loud-mouth is used to being the centre of attention, the life and soul of the party, they're not necessarily the most respected. Their very loudness can cheapen what they have to say.

When it comes to the aspie, they listen to everyone equally or not at all. The loudness of the loud-mouth can put them off at first so there is often some scenario, as described above, where they meet on common ground and have a chance to know each other. Once that has happened, they can be firm friends.

In return, the aspie is fascinated, bewitched at times, with how easily their friend moves through life. Why do people listen? How do they enjoy social occasions? Why can they always think of something to say? How do people laugh *with* them and not *at* them? The aspie may spend some time almost studying the loud-mouth, looking for their secret, as well as enjoying the novelty of watching their polar opposite drum through life.

The trouble can come when people with Aspergers have to mix in groups on a more regular basis and still can't make themselves heard. School and work would be the big examples here. At both, the aspie may be singled out, by boss or teacher, and asked a direct question. If the aspie can overcome their initial panic, the answer is probably forthcoming. They would still be viewed as non-communicative, though, because they had to be prompted.

What the aspie says may be sparkling but will count for little unless people pay attention. Just as a loud-mouth may be discounted for being over the top, the quiet aspie's persona will mean their words are tolerated, when heard. They are seen as too quiet, not pushy enough, no confidence. If someone is seen as having no confidence, how can you trust what they have to say?

They are often told to speak up, stand up, just say it, spit it out...The audience, if they do listen, will wear the familiar expressions of slight bemusement, tolerating what the aspie is saying until it's time to listen to someone who knows what they're talking about.

This is such a frustrating dilemma for many aspies and, naturally, means they often stop speaking up as there seems little point. Resentment can build, as they decide not to bother if people can't be bothered with them. This does nothing to resolve the issue, only making it worse.

The solution? Do we go under-cover and pretend to be the loud-mouth? I don't think we'd manage that very well. Sometimes by imagining yourself the loud-mouth, you can project some volume and veneer of confidence which helps a little.

I think the secret here is in finding out when it's good to speak and when it doesn't matter. If you find yourself in a group where you might as well be counting the seconds off, rather than being able to contribute verbally, then you're in the wrong group. If you really need to push yourself to the middle for them to take notice, are they the sort of people who need to be listening to you?

Seek out like-minded people and, even with little confidence, you'll find they are more willing to listen. If you are forced to interact with a group that's less receptive and it's important for you to be heard, break them up into real people and ask for help.

Choose a sympathetic person and explain your difficulties. If you need your voice to be heard, then there is more chance of people hearing two voices than one. And you might make a new friend along the way.

I would emphasise, groups that don't or can't listen to you aren't the right groups for you. I realise that sometimes they will be your own family (they can be the worst offenders) but it's still worth holding out for people who *want* to listen to you, who are truly interested in what you have to say.

You'll be surprised how your quiet voice, in the right place, with the right people, can be heard just as well as the loud ones. It's a feeling worth waiting for.

Truth and lies with an aspie on the side

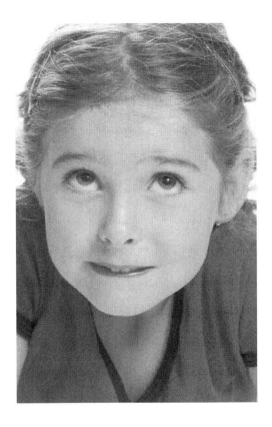

Let's be clear: by nature, aspies are stoutly honest. Often brutally, harshly, unflinchingly honest. If you ask them a straight question, you can bet the answer will come back fast enough to hit you between the eyes. That's just how it is and it's the big bonus and drawback of living in close proximity with Aspergers.

Now, replay that track a little and it soon becomes clear why an aspie would also be less than truthful and, over time, learn to lie to get themselves out of trouble. Some of us make quite good liars too, depending on the circumstances.

Let me explain.

If an aspie doesn't understand the question, you may get a wrong answer. If they were thinking about something else, you may get the wrong answer. If your question too strongly reminded them of sheep, your answer will be wool.

That's the simple side of Aspergers and honesty. Dishonesty usually only comes into play by accident. That leads us naturally to...

Those occasions when the truth doesn't work.

As a child with Aspergers, you are onto a losing streak when it comes to getting yourself out of trouble. If you do something wrong, and understand you have done something wrong, it won't occur to you to lie when asked about it.

If you do something wrong and don't understand it's wrong, or don't understand the question, then your answer won't match what the other person wants to hear, so you get accused of lying.

For example, you break the thing you were told not to touch. Except, you weren't told not to touch it - you were told to be *careful* with it. You *were* being careful with it, you held it very carefully and then, suddenly, you weren't holding it any more.

When the other person comes back to find a guilty looking child amongst the pieces of something which used to be whole, their first reaction will usually be anger, followed by the question: 'Why did you touch it?'

The conversation might follow these lines (assuming the mini-aspie isn't too shy to speak up).

Adult: Why did you touch it?

Mini-aspie: I wanted to hold it.

Adult: I told you not to touch it!

Mini-aspie shakes head.

Adult, becoming angrier: I told you not to touch it!!

Mini-aspie: No, you didn't.

Adult, infuriated, egged on by sight of broken pieces of beloved thing: 'How dare you lie to me!'

And so on, until the mini-aspie is convinced the adult has memory deficit disorder and the adult knows the mini-aspie can take responsibility for nothing and is willing to lie to cover their tracks.

You see, in the adult's mind, it's obvious when saying 'be careful with it', that they mean 'don't touch it'. To any child, but especially an aspie child, these aren't the same thing. Other children learn the connections between what is said and what is implied. They learn to marry up different phrases to mean the same thing.

So, 'it's hot,' 'it's too hot to eat' and 'be careful, it's hot' all come to mean that the food is too hot to eat right now and you need to blow on it before you try to eat it. To an aspie child, if you manage to catch them before they burn their mouth off shoving it in, you must say, 'blow on it before you eat it'. You can't go through the whole rigmarole of explaining it's hot so you must blow on it because they'll probably stop listening halfway through. They can see it's hot, there's steam coming off it!

And I think some of you may be working round to thinking that the aspie child will learn what those phrases mean when they burn their mouth off eating hot food; am I right? Yes, that would be nice. Except, when the mini-aspie does chew the hot chicken and burns their mouth off, the next time they are served hot chicken, or cold chicken, or luke-warm chicken, they won't eat it. Do you know why? Because chicken burns your mouth off.

Serve them hot beef or soup or porridge with steam rising in Gandalf-esque shapes towards the ceiling and they'll eat it right up - and, naturally, burn their mouths off.

If you don't step in (you cruel parent) and warn them about hot food, you may reach a stage where all they'll eat is cornflakes and crisps, and no one wants that.

I exaggerate slightly, as most adults would warn small children about hot food, even when it's served at a temperature that's quite safe to eat straight away. Another reason for me going over this is that aspies are very temperature sensitive a lot of the time, so something that is safe to eat for everyone else may feel too hot to them, and that means you'll still get the negative reaction re the chicken above.

So, forgive me the small diversion into literal descriptive language there; I wanted you to see how language is so very important with aspies, especially when it comes to them knowing what is expected and so learning how they can be honest all the time with you.

Back to when they were small and hardly anything made sense. If you have otherwise sane and loving adults who suddenly lose their tempers for no good reason, that can be very disconcerting. One minute you have a nice Granny who thinks you're fab and the next you hear her shouting at you from across the room because you left the cupboard open again and the dog ate a week's worth of dog food in two minutes.

You deny leaving it open, not because you know you should have closed it (you're not stupid), but because you can't remember leaving it open in the first place. Aspies forget things - a lot. The grandchild will remember they're always meant to close the cupboard. That important lesson will have gone in after the kerfuffle over the other times the dog ate a week's worth of food. What went wrong was that they became distracted this time and forgot they had left the cupboard open. That's not exactly the same thing as being wilfully naughty.

So they get told off for doing the bad thing again and this time they deny doing the bad thing. Granny, faced with yet more money down the drain (or down the dog), is furious, made worse by the denial of any wrongdoing. She checks the mini-aspie remembers about closing the cupboard. Yes, mini-aspie assures her, *of course* they remember about the cupboard. A row ensues, during which Granny is driven to heights of temper by the blank expression of her grandchild and the sound of the dog burping in the background.

At the end of all this, it becomes clear to Granny that mini-aspie is lying to get themselves out of trouble. What other explanation could there be? She knows mini-aspie is clever as anything and closing the cupboard is a very easy thing to do. You can't just forget to close a cupboard, not when you're standing right next to it and the dog has to push past you to steal the food!

Mini-aspie makes things worse by not owning up to the lie and insisting they have done nothing wrong. They can't remember how the cupboard came to be opened again. It must have been the dog!

After this, there is an issue of trust between Granny and mini-aspie. The kitchen becomes out of bounds until the grandchild learns responsibility and the dog has lost some weight. The next time Granny asks mini-aspie to do something, she will supervise and check and ask annoying questions to make sure the thing is done. This leads to more arguments.

Eventually, trust will build, the grandchild will be secure once more and all will be fine - until mini-aspie forgets to do something, or misunderstands and denies all knowledge of simple instructions. And away we go again.

It is very, very difficult to explain to a non-aspie how something simple and immediate can be forgotten so completely. I don't really blame them for thinking it is lying and nothing else. It doesn't make sense for someone to forget the thing they were just talking about. How can it slip the mind in so little time?

Given enough instances of this kind of row and getting into trouble, the growing aspie will dread being given things to do. For all the times it goes right, there will be a humdinger of a time when it goes wrong. It's the hot chicken all over again.

As the aspie ages, they learn a little of what people want and expect when trouble flares. They learn pretty quickly that what they do not want is a gormless expression, shoulder shrugging, a hapless smile and an 'I forgot'. They certainly, definitely, absolutely *hate* it beyond any rational limit, if you relay back to them exactly what they said and how they said it, showing the aspie wasn't in the wrong after all. As far as non-aspies are concerned, a failure to understand the instructions within the instructions (*be careful, it's hot* meaning the same as *blow on it before you eat it*), is as bad as not listening to the instructions at all. In fact, it's the same as **doing it on purpose**!

Fast forward to your adult aspie and they've been in the doghouse so often they've chosen curtains and a new rug to make it seem like home. So when they get into trouble, their natural honesty has been pushed aside and subverted into a need to give people the answer they want. It's not lying so much as fitting in.

As an adult aspie, if you break the precious thing because you held it when you weren't supposed to, you won't explain you forgot or say you misunderstood. You'll see instantly that you've done it again and you need to stop the other person from being upset. You'll say something on the spur of the moment, like I tripped and fell against it, or I thought it had a crack so wanted to check.

To be honest, most excuses and fake answers will be pretty lame and not very convincing and so the mistrust and belief in the aspie's dishonesty grows. Your reputation for not being able to explain yourself and give a straight answer is stronger than ever. And still, when the other option is to say, honestly, 'I'm sorry, it looked so nice and I forgot I wasn't supposed to touch it,' you know the person wouldn't accept that as the truth either. By lying, you run the risk of being disbelieved but you also aim for those times when you achieve the goal and make the person less upset. Telling the truth never seems to stop them being upset and it becomes the lesser option.

This view of aspie honesty/dishonesty is important for anyone dealing with aspies of any age, but I'll direct this last part to people living with the adult versions. The adult with Aspergers has had many years of trying to save feelings and avoid upsetting scenes and noisy arguments. They come to you as a made thing, a creation of their upbringing and their experience, where truth has so often equalled trouble. If you ask them a good, honest question about something they did not affect, like whether your new hairstyle looks good - then you'll get an uncompromising and honest answer or a sad little smile as they try to be kind (which is almost the same thing).

The difference comes when the question relates to something *they* have done wrong, or even *feel* they have done wrong. Then you should listen a little more carefully to the answer and see if any translation is necessary. If you really want the truth about what happened to Aunt Ivy's prize cockerel, you shouldn't ask, 'What happened? What did you do?' Instead try something more forgiving like, 'Did something go wrong? Do you need my help?' A gentler form of questioning may bring the right response.

If not, you'll just have to learn to translate and show your aspie in word and deed that they are safe with you, that the truth is also safe with you and help them return to that clear, clean feeling of never having to say the wrong thing again.

Aspies are still liars...

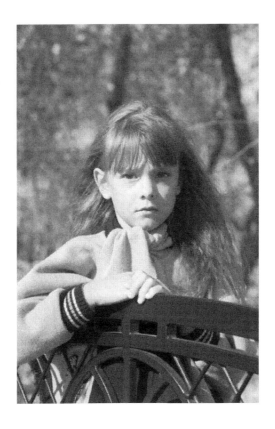

Ever since I started my aspie blog, people have found it by searching 'aspies' and 'lying', along with the expected variations like 'are all aspies liars', 'lying aspies' and 'dishonest aspies'.

Lots of people are dishonest and lots of people lie - and aspies are people, you know. So, before I defend anyone, better to ask if your particular aspie is a liar, rather than do all aspies lie. But yes, I know what you mean.

It can come across as lying, can't it? The evasive look, not meeting your eye; the inability to commit or to answer your questions in the way you expect. The strange, complicated conversation you have when you try to talk about something really important and come away with a new recipe for brownies instead.

We can be very. very evasive. I admit it, I can evade with the best of them, from avoiding any eye contact at all to actually fleeing the scene. It's all just part of the fight or flight reaction, and aspies FLY.

If I think you'll want me to have a heavy, in-depth talk about the state of our relationship, I'm flapping those wings before you've finished the first sentence. If I suspect more is wanted of me than I am willing or able to give, I take a look around in case I need to run before I can launch.

If I'm confused as to what someone actually wants, and I'm worried about it; then it makes much more sense to flap off in another direction and wait for things to feel normal again before I show my face.

It's not lying, it's *evasion* and the difference is in the intention. Liars set out with a deliberate intent to deceive, often for their own gain. Evasive aspies just want life to be uncomplicated and to be able to move onto the next stage without having to work out the perils of this one.

Evasion and lying are like two small children in kindergarten. They both took a cookie from the tray before the teacher told them to. The liar took it and lied because he wanted that cookie and he was ready for it now. The evasive aspie took it because she was passing and saw cookies and hadn't the teacher said they were all going to have cookies later? Was now later?

Having discovered now was not later, she becomes the evasive aspie, keen to get out of the latest trouble with no real clue as to how she got into it in the first place.

The trouble is, lying and evasion often end in the same way, with someone looking at you as if they're disappointed and you feeling like a big problem.

Lying and aspies may lead you to Asperger blogs online but don't let the same search take you the wrong way when it comes to your own aspie. Make sure you know the difference between deceit and confusion, between subterfuge and fear. They may look the same from a distance but take a closer look and with less anger in your heart.

We are only people, in the end, and so are you.

7: Real Communication

So, now we get to the heart of it – real communication. I don't mean complete opening up or even a full explanation of feelings and motivations; I believe real communication can be as simple as a touch of the hand.

Real communication, full and honest without barriers, is the goal in any relationship and can seem further away in relations with an aspie. We are constrained by how we feel, by what we have learned and mostly by how we struggle to express ourselves. When you fight to be open with others it is no surprise that you have an even bigger battle to find the right words to express yourself.

I truly relish those times when I meet a person who seems to understand me and who can be counted as a friend without me feeling like I am giving too much away. Relationships are often fraught and difficult, yet for each of these there are those in life who make it all better, the ones who can reach out and listen without you having to say anything.

Readers, this section is for all those times when we aspies, usually at the mercy of our own barriers, finally feel at home with a person. We may not show it, we may never express it but the feeling will be there.

Sometimes true communication can be painful, too, as the aspie opens up a little further than you expected and lets you know what is on their mind – at length and in great detail. Too much disclosure is annoyingly at odds with not expressing ourselves but at least it means life with an aspie is never dull!

If your aspie feels comfortable enough to tell you how you look in your new outfit or tell your mother how she looks in hers or explain what happened to the vase you were given last Christmas or moan endlessly about the noise from the heating system or even to scream and shout and slam all the doors in the house in a fury on their way to a safe place, then you should take it as a compliment. Your aspie may be hard to live with at times but by letting go and being too expressive, you know you are part of the safe place.

Here's to real communication, whether it is words or only a look shared as we pass on our way through life.

Bluntness or Honesty?

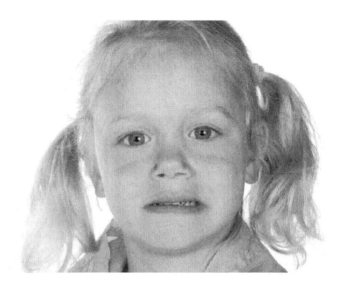

IT Teen had been told by a friend that he was as blunt as a butter knife, which made me laugh until IT revealed he had replied by saying, "If I'm as blunt as a butter knife then my mother is as blunt as its wooden handle."

"I'm not that bad!" I cried, picturing the offending knife with an unwieldy, rustic handle, not so much spreading the butter as flattening it into the table.

"Yes, you are," IT replied. "I didn't even think I *was* blunt before now, because I always compared myself to you!"

So, the acerbic, brutally honest, psychological enema that is IT Teen thought he wasn't even blunt?? I thought of all the times his essential bluntness has risen to the surface like a basking shark. Then I thought about myself.

If IT Teen, that bastion of bluntness, thinks I am the handle to his knife, what do I do to people? I know I can say the wrong thing and am overly honest, but if IT cuts to the core with the things he says, what do *I* do?

This is a terrifying concept, readers. It makes me feel open to the elements, left on the mountain tops with only one foot on the path. I feel buffeted, blown backwards towards the scree, helpless to hold onto anything solid as the weather closes in and the clouds meld with the land.

All those times when I've blurted the truth, have I been emotionally sand-blasting the other person? Has their silence or quiet agreement been a stunned response? How many times have I hurt instead of helped?

So, I talked about it with RT Teen, himself something of an aspie honesty monster. He's less blunt than IT, if you count bluntness and honesty as two separate things. He also was aghast at the idea of anyone being blunter than IT but did snigger at me being a handle.

We talked about the idea that what we considered helpful honesty was, in all truth, nothing but bluntness in a different light. We hesitantly admitted that our honest answers may have been felt and seen in the same way as IT's pickaxe approach.

We came to the conclusion that perhaps honesty becomes bluntness in the telling: that letting it fall out of you, without hesitation, into the middle of a normal conversation, turns vital honesty into blunt endeavour. That perhaps it's all in the telling, after all, with the tone of voice, or expression, making an honest response a more harmful one.

Then, never one to let honesty fall to the wayside, I said to RT Teen,

"You know, this is all very well but maybe people just call honesty bluntness because they don't want to hear the truth?"

He thought for a second, then agreed happily. We came away from this worrying debate solid in our beliefs once again.

Honesty is still for the best, even if other, gentler souls call it bluntness. Honesty has a true face that aspies see and name. It becomes other words to other people because they are so used to operating in a world that expects one person to behave differently in so many situations. If we could all simply be ourselves, all the way through, then honesty would always be recognised.

I do feel I may be excusing myself rather lightly here. I know I am an awful, terrible, frightening teller-of-the-truth. I know it upsets people. And I do, really, really do wish, I could be more tactful a lot of the time.

I hate it when my big, honest mouth lands me in it or I hurt someone - *especially* when I hurt someone. I get tired of other people having to think to themselves, 'She doesn't mean it that way, she's only being direct'. I would like to be eloquent more often.

And yet, I do feel I would rather have it this way. Let other people have their belief that honesty has many different faces. I like to see things as they actually are, without a veil between. I like to know the real answers to every question.

Honesty, bluntness, directness, tactlessness - call them what you will, I have the complete set in original boxes and I know their worth. I see the world in a certain way and they help me to explain it to you.

If I sometimes say the wrong thing, or more likely, the right thing that you would rather not hear, then I apologise. I'm confident in the knowledge that I'm unable to see it any other way and that it's usually better to have clarity between us than kindly-meant subterfuge.

Oh, and readers, one more thing. Without that big, blunt handle, you wouldn't be able to use the butter knife. And without the butter knife, you would have dry toast with no butter! Faced with such a dreadful alternative, it's always better to have the use of a good, solid handle between you and the toast.

How to talk to non-aspies: 1

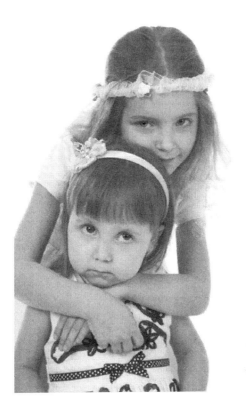

So many people find my blog and books by searching 'how to talk to aspies'. It struck me as much more useful to learn how to talk to non-aspies, as it's something so many of us struggle with.

Non-aspies hold positions of great power, in society and in our lives. They are the coping ones, the managing, the holding down the job, two kids, mortgage and small pottery business while we aspies struggle to manage the new tap on the bathroom sink, let alone going out to conquer the universe.

Talking to non-aspies can be complicated as they often want to know things but have a very poor way of expressing themselves. It is the non-aspie who needs to know what you find difficult about the new tap and learning how to tell them, in ways they will understand, can seem like an uphill struggle.

When they ask why the bathroom is flooded, we tell them the new tap did it. Of course, the tap had an aspie attached to it at the time, so the non-aspie will try again: Why did we flood the bathroom?

At this point it's very tempting to wonder (perhaps out loud) if the non-aspie is stoopid. I mean, we already told them the tap is to blame. Obviously! But what the non-aspie is looking for is the reason why we, the attachee of the tap, managed to flood the bathroom again.

They want to know what we did, you see. They want to find out how it is possible for an intelligent person to not be able to use a tap simply because it is different from the old one. And also, while we're at it, they want to know why we left the tap on long enough for the bathroom to flood.

Instead of asking these things, they ask why we flooded the bathroom. This implies a level of blame we simply refuse to recognise. The tap is at fault, the water from the tap flooded the bathroom. Our presence in the vicinity has little to do with these facts; it could have happened to anyone (it's always us, though).

Don't ask me why non-aspies prefer to speak in code instead of just going for the real questions. I think perhaps they have some kind of social awareness issue, where they expect others to guess what they are thinking without having to say it. They maybe think we are all on some giant psychic pulse where we know the insides of their heads like the insides of the biscuit barrel.

So, when speaking to non-aspies I suggest you keep it simple. They like answers, even though they often claim we give the wrong ones. Try asking them what they want to know and see if that clears it up more quickly. Rather than guessing what they want, say something like, 'Did you want to know why the bathroom flooded?'

As we've discovered, they want to know *why* we flooded the bathroom, so turning the question around is likely to get their attention, even if they appear a little agitated at having it returned to sender.

Once you have their attention, do not abuse this privilege by asking them how they expect you to cope with a new tap when they know full well you don't read instructions. And don't moan on about how much better the old tap was when you know it leaked for two years. Try asking them to watch you use the blasted thing and see if you can figure out why it keeps flooding the bathroom.

You see, talking to non-aspies does involve focus and dedication on the part of the aspie. It's always worth repeating what they have said to see if you have it right and then keeping your calm when they lose theirs. This method does work in the end and means you will both be focused on the questions that matter rather than spending half an hour of your precious time waiting for the non-aspie to figure out which question they really like.

In the end, talking to non-aspies requires patience and some foresight. Keep in mind their habit of dodging the real questions and try to make them hone their attention so you can help them understand what you are saying.

Remember, they always assume you know exactly what they mean, regardless of the many times you failed this test before. And they haven't yet figured out not everyone is psychic.

(How to talk to non-aspies: 2 is in the Guides section at the end of the book).

The politeness balloon

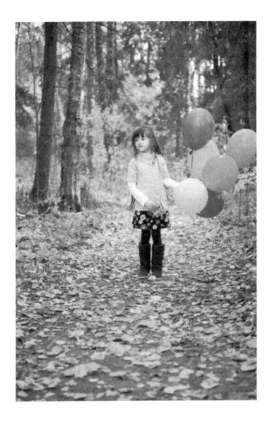

Sometimes I wish everyone was as direct as an aspie. For all the times we miss the point and get it wrong and say the worst thing that comes into our heads, we spare people the run-around of a pointless conversation-loop.

I have just had one of those infuriating conversations with a non-aspie where they have a specific *thing* they want to know. They have it right there, sitting up-front in the big boy chair, waiting to be seen and answered. So, what do they do?

Rather than be honest and find out what they want to know, I am subjected to a mind-numbing exchange of questions and hum-herm-ah comments where my answers to the questions obviously aren't hitting the mark.

That's the funny thing about not asking a direct question, though - you don't tend to get a direct answer!

Am I meant to know what is behind the questions? Or am I meant to be seduced by politeness and then somehow have the real questions revealed to me? Am I happier, now that we have gone all around the houses, back out the side gate and down the lane to Aunty Joan's before getting to the right answer? Do I sound happy??

If this conversation had been with an aspie, it would have taken a few seconds.

Aspie 1: 'Oh yeah - hang on, my shoe lace has done that thing I hate - there! Now, what time are we getting back from Mars on Friday?'

Aspie 2: 'Probably about five, I have to detour to Pluto to pick up my new hum-a-bing.'

Aspie 1: 'Great! I need to be back before six so that's perfect.'

There, wasn't that easy? No one was hurt, it took no time at all and we even had a few extra seconds for re-tying shoelaces. Isn't life simple when you ask the question that is really in your mind, instead of all the little questions that are meant to make life softer?

Of course, I am being generous to aspies. I know that half the time the aspie wouldn't ask the question and only remember they needed to be back by six when we were still trying to get out of the Mars car park at five-thirty. But, in general, if aspies are not distracted by the shoelace and if they remember to speak in the first place, then a direct question will be asked - and answered.

Now, non-aspies, please, I beg of you, take it on trust that we are unlikely to be hurt or discomfited by a direct question. It is the jigging around with the politeness balloon that drives us absolutely crazy. Really, it does. Be offensive if you like, but be quick about it and be honest. Then we can all get on with our lives!

The moaning aspie

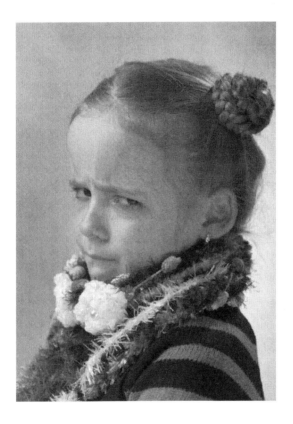

Picture it. You finally get your aspie out of the house and into the car. After a morning of torment, you are on your way to great aunt Veronica's house and only an hour late! What an effort it's been, what a super-human feat it seemed at seven a.m. when you had to wake the aspie and make them get out of bed. Between then and now you have proven yourself a supremo of aspie handling. With your skills in diplomacy and tricky situations, you should join the United Nations!

For a moment, for a brief, blessed second, you smile to yourself in the car. At last, mission accomplished: off to dear old Veronica's house and this time you didn't leave your aspie behind.

Then it starts. A small noise perhaps, a little complaint. The seat belt won't come undone, the seat belt won't work properly, the seat belt is somehow already looped around your aspie's shoulder. Seat belt tamed you drive on, determined this is going to work.

The favourite CD isn't in the car, the window is open and the wind is blowing their hair. The vent will let in smells that insult the aspie nasal experience. The window, the big, sheer, uncompromising windscreen is letting in too much light and where did those sunglasses go?

There is a slight moment of rest where the aspie gathers themselves and looks out of the side window… then it starts again. A fidget, a shuffle, a movement suggestive of one lone ant in the pants, just the one, just enough to set the aspie moving in their seat. Sometimes that lone ant is joined by more, other times the attention flicks back to the radio, or the fact they forgot to charge their phone and the battery is bound to die before they even reach Aunt Veronica's and what on earth are they meant to do for the whole visit as did you know that Aunt Veronica doesn't even have a computer?!

Another moment of peace as the aspie pauses to reflect on this astounding fact. No computer and not even any internet! Maybe not even a mobile phone!

That ant is back, the shoes are involved this time and the feet are trudging about in the foot well as if the ground is hot beneath them. Why can they never get comfortable in the car? Why can't we get a bigger car? Why is it so sunny? And why did they have to come?

Eventually you reach this question, the same question they have launched at you since they found out you expected them to leave the house and visit with Veronica. Why do you need them to come? Why could you not go on your own? You went the last two times on your own so why not this time?

By this stage you will have exhausted all logical discussion on the matter. You will have explained that it looks bad if you always visit alone, that Aunt Veronica likes to see her nephew, that you are tired of going places on your own all the time, that it will not kill the aspie to leave the house and the computer just occasionally seeing as you don't ask them to do much, do you?!

Sullen silence followed logical discussion and your aspie could see no way out of the visit, driven this time by guilt at avoiding elderly Veronica as well as letting you down. Grudging acceptance of the visit crept in and by bedtime of the night before, you knew your aspie would be coming with you. At last!

That does not mean it is over, though. The journey to Aunt Veronica's will be full of unseen ants and hot floors and evil seat belts and mysteriously absent CDs and an untuneable radio and all manner of annoyances which make it very clear the aspie should have stayed home today. Like signs and portents, these little irritations will take over the aspie consciousness and impress upon them that they were right to want to stay at home. And they would have stayed at home, if you hadn't made them come out!

Like travellers who have journeyed so far their suffering is etched into their faces, you finally arrive at Veronica's house. The old lady is very pleased to see you both and your aspie is brought into the warmth of a family visit. For now, the moaning is over, though watch out for the rolling eyes and the sighing and hoffing and scratching and general discomfort of being somewhere so unconducive to aspie life.

Now all you have to do is get home again, with your aspie worn out by this being-social business and just desperate to get back to where they belong. Of course, having used massive amounts of energy today they will probably get nothing at all done once they are home. Imagine the progress they might have made if you hadn't forced them to come!

Turn up the untuneable radio or put in your favourite CD for a change (be prepared to growl when the aspie hand reaches out to change it) and congratulate yourself that you made the visit happen and that, for the next two times, you can leave that aspie at home again and have a nice trip by yourself.

Nobody moans like an aspie

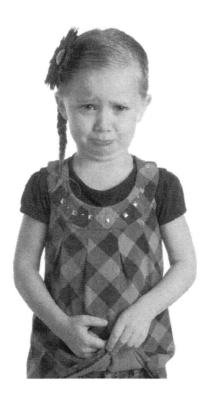

I'm insulting myself here. Perhaps all other aspies are paragons of quiet sufferance and never utter a word against their circumstances? Perhaps I am the only moaner?

I don't think so, somehow. I think moaning is one of those aspects of aspie-hood that doesn't get mentioned in official circles but is talked about an awful lot amongst people who have to live with us. How many times has the parent of an aspie held off from doing something that would upset their child, not simply because it would be upsetting but more due to the unending, self-perpetuating, dripping mooooooaaaaannnnn? I know I have.

When RT Teen was a mini-RT he had no problems holding conversations. What he did have a problem with was other people butting in before he'd finished. It seemed worse in the car as mini-IT Teen was incredibly fond of butting in, so the two of them together were a nightmare to travel with.

RT would start to tell us something and he'd spend time getting the words out. A bit like a mental stutter, he hesitated within his sentences as he thought of the next part, then he would bring out finely crafted phrases. All of this was lost on little IT who would rail, 'Just say it! Say it!'

Being interrupted always had the opposite effect as mini RT would then stop, go back to the start of his sentence and begin again. He never forgot the words which came before and repeated this process until he was able to say the whole thing without one interruption.

Over time, mini IT and myself learned to sit, rigid, while mini RT told us things. Even a noise or a tut would be enough to stop him and make it all repeat. And then it became like a moan as he repeated and repeated what he wanted to say.

So, he wasn't moaning as such but his repetition and constant need to speak without interruption were like a moan, as they were a reaction to what was going on around him and what he perceived as other people being difficult with him.

In general, if anything went wrong, normally cheerful mini RT would groan and grumble, flopping about as if he had weights on his shoulders. He would either make many different sounds which meant nothing, but together made a moan, or he would set up a wailing about the injustice of the situation and go on about it endlessly.

I have to admit, I was just as bad as a child. Worse, in fact, as I kept it going for much longer but with less drama. My mother and step-father were very fond of hill-walking (the inhumanity!) and as they both worked full-time, I'd be dragged out at the weekends, over yet more sodden Lake District fell tops.

I hated those walks with a passion. What I actually wanted to do with my weekends was stay at home and read, but apparently I could read anytime and I should be enjoying the beautiful scenery and appreciating how lucky I was to live near such a wonderful place.

I used to beg them to leave me in the car while they went on the walk. And the backpack always felt so heavy, digging into my shoulders and seeming like a pointless punishment in itself.

Those boots, those rotten, brown, laced boots, they never protected me from anything. If there was a deep puddle or a bog, I ended up in it and it just went right over the top of the boots. And they were so hot! Having to wear thick socks with them didn't help. Sometimes, the boots were what I hated the most of all.

No, what I really hated was seeing the backs of my parents as they strode off ahead of me on the path with me coming along behind, feeling all my troubles cluster as I struggled through life. They would wait at the top of the hill and be rested when I got there, then leap up as soon as I arrived and carry on going. The unfairness!

I moaned from start to finish on those walks. I really don't know why they bothered taking me. If I was them, I'd have left me behind. I don't know how much enjoyment they gained with me following along behind like a little rain cloud, drip, drip, drip with my moaning.

Everything was wrong and I would never enjoy it and they knew I didn't enjoy it, so why take me? And not everybody liked walking and I was never going to like it just because they did. I could think of many things I'd rather be doing and didn't they care that I was upset? Didn't they care that my feet were too hot and I had blisters and my backpack was heavier than theirs?

And so on. Until, by the end of the walk, the sighs of relief had more to do with me shutting up when I saw the car than completing their trek. Me, back in the comfort of a man-made environment, could at last take up my book or gaze, unseeing, at the landscape outside the windows.

Now that I'm grown up, I know I moan and I do try not to. I honestly do! But it's just the way things are and a good moan can be very therapeutic. Sometimes you need to get it all off your chest, even if the person listening to you feels like pouring breakfast all over your head. Sometimes, you just can't stop.

I've had poor IT Teen wriggle and gyrate in the car, trapped with myself and RT Teen as we're both setting up a-moaning. He loses his temper and tells us off, asking why we have to moan all the time anyway? He points out that what we're moaning about is not important, it's not worth us going on.

That usually ends badly as I sit there in a sulk, thinking that I wasn't even moaning while with RT the tinderbox of injustice is lit and he's telling IT why his moaning is *not* moaning, it's complaining, which is different, because he's being reasonable about whatever it was that went wrong. At which point a full-scale argument ensues and I have to threaten them with dire consequences if they don't quiet down and let me drive.

After a brief silence, RT will always be the first to speak, adding a small moan to encapsulate the much larger one he had been going through before and then IT turns a funny colour and starts gyrating again.

You see, that's the other thing with aspie moans: as well as being pretty much endless once we've started, we have to have the last word. Come on, you know it's true. Even if the last word is a slammed door, a kicked wall, a growl or a broken pencil, that word will be had.

We have to put our point across, one way or another, and if we feel the need to moan then we'll either do just that or find some other way to get it out of the system.

Readers, I won't sugar-coat it: being a moany bunch does not endear aspies but it is a good way of getting our troubles out there, even if we end up moaning about something other than what is really bothering us.

Much better to have the dripping of the moan than the inflammatory meltdown or physical reaction to stress. Better to have the voice droning on in your ear than to have it raised in temper or anguish.

Honestly, I know when it comes to sticking plasters that a quick rip is better than a slow tear but when it comes to the aspie in full flow, a slow moan is better than an explosive tantrum.

And you can trust me, I've tried both.

Understanding the tone of voice

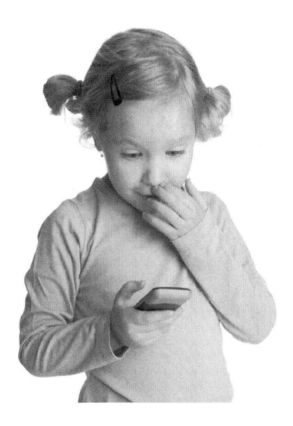

I had a Tone of Voice inflicted on me yesterday. Luckily, it came with a set of instructions on what I was meant to do with it so I didn't have to guess what I'd done wrong or how I had been a terrible person - this time.

How many times do other people use tones of voice to get their message across without a set of instructions though? I've been subjected to seemingly normal sentences delivered in a sorrowful/angry/irritated/name-your-poison tone of voice which made no sense in relation to what was being said.

I believe this comes under the heading of 'but you should *know*'.

For instance, we may be having a conversation about where to go for lunch and the words would follow what I was expecting, such as what time, where to meet, where to have lunch and who else is coming along. All of this might be normal.

Replay this conversation with the other person using a short, huffy tone, as though you just ate their last chocolate or kicked their mother's behind and it stops making sense. It becomes a very awkward conversation as I am answering questions and replying to the right things but the other person's tone of voice suggests there is another agenda.

I have found that when people behave this way they either want me to notice so I can be the one who 'starts' it by asking what's wrong or, maddeningly, they don't want to discuss what is wrong but do expect me to know what I've done.

Readers, life is short enough and tiring enough without having to play this pointless guessing game, especially when the reason behind the latest tone of voice turns out to be something we were completely unaware of or an innocent mistake.

As an aspie of long-standing social clumsiness, I am used to being in the wrong and being to blame for things but that doesn't mean I instinctively know each time what I have done. Sometimes, no matter how angry or sorrowful the tone of voice, I still don't know. And just occasionally I haven't done anything at all!

So I would like people to do what I have often requested and **just spit it out**. Tell me the problem, lay it in front of me and let me look at it. Let's talk about it like grown-ups and not behave like a small child who needs persuading to do what is good for them.

Life is so much easier if we just use the tone of voice to match the words we are speaking at the time and not the tone of voice to match the internal monologue which, to be honest, no one else can hear.

Getting the wrong end of the stick...and waving it

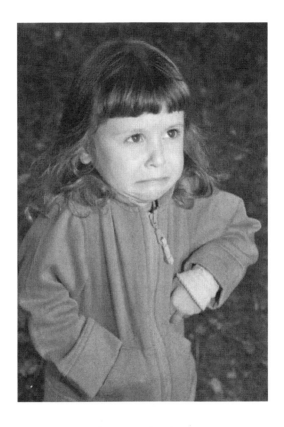

In other words, taking something completely the wrong way or misunderstanding what your own senses are telling you. It's very easily done and can cause great confusion.

A small example: I was sitting in my car when I heard a man whistling, the kind you do to get someone's attention. He kept repeating it and I was looking to see where he was. A few seconds later I spotted him. It was an older gent in a bright pink jacket with a shopping bag. He was moving along the pavement at speed, doing a jig as he went. He was bent slightly as he jigged, laughing, and was focused on the man walking ahead of him, who seemed oblivious to being followed.

The older man was speeding up and would soon reach his target. He had his head lower now and if he didn't slow down, he'd barrel right into the back of the man in front. I waited to see what would happen, wondering if he was going to jump on him or head butt him or even hit him with the carrier bag. Whatever, he certainly looked like he was having fun.

Then, at the last second, the man in front crossed the road and the older gent's target was revealed to be a woman waiting at the very end of the road, patiently watching him do his jig as he came towards her. He slowed in front of her, still laughing and gave her a little bow, then the shopping bag.

Everything he had done was for her. He had whistled to get her attention then entertained her with his running jig. He never had any interest in the innocent man walking in front of him and, luckily, the man didn't hear him or look behind at the wrong moment.

All became clear, this time, and it made sense. If I had looked past the man in front I might have seen the woman and understood but once I had in my mind the scenario I thought was right, I stopped looking for another explanation. As far as I was concerned, the older gent was about to spring some kind of surprise on the other man and even though this behaviour was out of the ordinary, it still never occurred to me to look for a different answer.

It's a small example of how wrong you can be, or at least how wrong *I* can be. I mean, why would a gentleman of a certain age jig along the pavement to jump on a stranger? Is it not more rational that I had missed a detail and he had a good reason for acting as he did? Does this mean I see it as more reasonable, in my own world view, for him to do something odd than something normal?

I tend to think people behave oddly a lot of the time and they're not really doing anything extraordinary; it's just they seem odd to me. This makes it easier to accept odd behaviour when it happens, as it doesn't seem very different from what is classed as normal behaviour by most people.

I often find myself hesitating and trying to re-think, in case I'm wrong. It causes an annoying type of hesitation which aggravates other people. If someone's behaviour seems perplexing to me, am I to ignore it and pretend I'm not confused or risk annoying the other person by seeking an explanation? Which way is best?

I've asked before, brought up what someone has done as it seems very relevant to the conversation at the time, only to be greeted with absolute disbelief that I would interrupt what was being said to ask about something a small child would understand. Standing, waiting for it to make sense while the other person waits to see if I'm serious.

Yes, I'm serious, even if that conversation was the wrong place to ask or this situation has nothing to do with my confusion. I do want to know why a person did this when it made no sense. No, it didn't make sense, not to me. No, I don't know why. No, I'm not just trying to change the subject.

It's a confusing mess at times, never improved by seeing the world in a different way so that even if you see it the right way today, you still doubt yourself tomorrow. But it does make life much more *interesting*, you know.

It doesn't really matter whether or not I have the wrong end of the stick; I'll carry on seeing things as they appear to be, only realising they are not what they seem later, when I've made the day a little stranger, funnier or more complicated.

It's much less boring to believe that a happy looking gent is about to surprise a stranger than to see the reality of an unimpressed woman watching him jive along the pavement. She may not have appreciated his antics, but I did. So, gent in the pink coat, I salute you for not caring whether the other man saw you and dancing anyway.

We should all do our own thing, readers, whether or not we have it wrong. In the end, we can only be ourselves and let other people worry about it if they will.

The eternal teenager

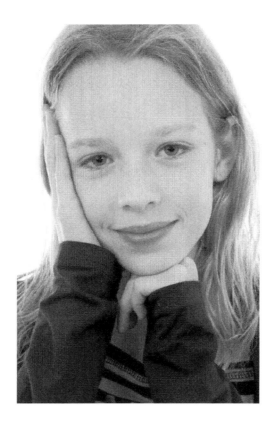

I freely admit to being stuck in my teens. Depending on the day, I can be anything from 13 to 15. On a good day I make it all the way to 17 and if it's a bad day I feel as old as 19, with the whole world to worry over.

The thing about teenagers is, in a normal family situation they are just getting ready to be fully fledged adults. They can take care of themselves in a lot of ways. They won't starve if you leave them alone, they know to lock the doors at night and feed the cat if it meows. They can do a job of work and be pretty much reliable.

They are emotionally volatile at times, ready to fly off the handle at a perceived wrong and also ready to support their friends no matter what. Your average teen can spin through a range of emotions in the same hour and come out the other end smiling.

They are creative and interested in doing fun things with their time. They know the value of free time and are not yet tied to the world of work and responsibility. They plan and hope and dream and understand that the world is an infinite place, made finite only by the adults who claim ownership over it.

Does any or all of this sound familiar? The aspie at large can identify with many teenage traits, not least of which is the belief that responsibility is a limited thing, not a constant companion and something to be treated with disdain if it gets too close.

When all's said and done, the emotions of the aspie which are close to the teenage world of feelings can be written off as being moody, difficult, hyper or over-sensitive. Lots of adults are capable of fulfilling these labels and more. But what brings the aspie closer to the teenager is that these emotions feel very natural, as if that's the way it's meant to be.

Proper grown up adults know, in moments of calm, that they shouldn't be moody, difficult, hyper and so on. Aspies look back and accept that those feelings were felt and believed in at the time and cannot be wished away.

When someone calls an aspie childish or melodramatic, besides it causing more arguments, it changes nothing. The aspie often knows they're being this way but that doesn't mean they can stop it. Like a teenager, they have greater self-awareness than a child but a limited ability to control their emotions and behaviour.

The attachment to friends is a very real aspect of the aspie as an eternal teenager. Most teens will do just about anything for their friends. At this stage in life, friends can become like family, understanding you in a way no one has before. It is now you realise there are other people in the world who you can choose to spend time with and who make what you are seem like a glorious thing.

Your friends don't tell you off, they don't want you to behave or change. They accept you as you are and celebrate you as a person. They are friends with you simply because they like you, not as an accident of genetics or because they have to share a house with you.

Friends *choose* you and an aspie who has been chosen is someone who knows the value of another person seeing them as they really are and actively seeking their company.

As responsibility to the silly things in life, like work and money, are shunned by the eternal teen, so are the responsibilities of friendship appreciated and respected. If the boss needs you on your day off it is a physical pain to go in and not be able to relax at home or do what you had planned. If your boss needs you on a proper work day but your friend also needs you, then you call in sick or flake off and go to your friend instead.

Teenagers eventually need to grow up and learn how to live in the real, adult world. The aspie eternal teen never really made this step. They saw the value of the world they discovered growing up, the one where they were finally left alone to do their own thing and realised the joy of obsessions and interests which would carry them through life.

Aspies know that the final step to being a grown up, someone who will live fully in the real world and accept everything that goes with that, is a hard one to take and fraught with danger. Aspies often try to take that extra step and find themselves tripping along an unknown path, with no way off the road and the feeling that they need to walk faster and faster just to get where they're going before the darkness comes.

Better to live as a teenager instead, with limited resources, not enough money and a shaky grip on responsibility, than to try to survive as an adult and see yourself fail at crucial moments. Aspies know there are things that need to be done, things which require an adult to do them. Sometimes it works and they can operate all the way up to their real age. Mostly it seems as if the trials of life are sent as a test of how successfully the aspie can avoid and hide from the nasties of a grown up world.

Being an eternal teenager is not ideal - far from it on many occasions! But it beats trying to live a lie, trying to succeed in a life that doesn't belong to you and which will never fully make sense. Sometimes, accepting who you are is a matter of also accepting *where* you are, in life and within yourself.

For me, I live as an eternal teenager, hopeful for the future and with the kind of self-knowledge that suggests, while anything is possible, I only have to do what is right for me. Of course, this isn't always true but like a real teenager I prefer to ignore that reality and make one of my own.

Living in your own reality is not a very grown up thing to do but it is surprisingly liberating. And readers, if it works most of the time then why not do it your way?

8: Guides

How are aspies awkward? Let me count the ways.

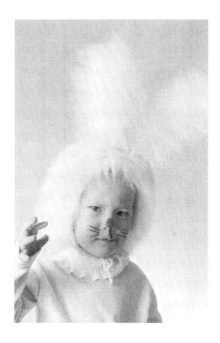

Actually, shall I just count the ways we're not awkward instead? It would be a lot quicker and might come across as more positive? Or am I just being awkward now?

All right then, but this list is not my final decision and I'm sure if you asked a non-aspie, then the awkwardness list would become an epic fantasy novel with dragons, battle-hardened maidens, songs around camp-fires, sprites in jars, no toilet facilities and too much protein.

The aspie is awkward in their physical attitude

We droop, we mooch, we bump into things, we get in the way, we trip over thin air, we drop stuff, we touch the TV and the house falls into darkness. If there is an awkward way to do something, we don't need to find it, it finds *us*.

Even aspies who are good with their hands will open the door the wrong way going into the shop, let it fall back accidentally against the little old lady then step on her as they turn back, trying to put things right.

The dog will be let loose as the lead slips through the fingers, the knife will chop the thumb and not the cheese, cleaning the toilet will always end badly, emptying the bin will mean cleaning the floor.

The aspie is awkward on the inside too

I don't understand, I misunderstand, I say whatever comes into my head, I tell you what I really think, I find something funny at the wrong moment, I cry at sad adverts, I don't cry when I'm supposed to, I thought you wanted me to do this?

282

I feel sad at precisely the wrong moment, I feel happy when you need empathy, I forget something important and remember every detail of last night's Hoarders. I thought you wanted my honest opinion?

Awkward decisions

It seemed like a good idea at the time, it made perfect sense, I didn't think of that, I thought you'd enjoy it, I didn't think you wanted it any more, I forgot it was worth that much money, I gave it to the dog, I cancelled, I paid before checking, I wanted it to be a surprise, I thought you liked cats, I never said I was a hairdresser.

Awkward lifestyle

I don't do crowds, I need my own space, I don't need much money, I've forgotten to pay the bills, I love this job, I've quit, I've become a vegetarian, I have allergies, it's not clean enough, but I *can* see the germs! I can't leave the house, I'll live in the attic, I can't, I have to go to Comic Con, I'm living as a wizard now.

Awkward obsessions

I love this, I'm sharing it with you, I'm sharing it with him too, I'm sharing it with the person next to me on the bus, I'm sharing it online, I'm sharing it with anyone who'll listen...What? That old thing? No, that's history, I love something else now. I'll share it with you!

Awkward finances

I have no money, I'll work it out, I'll be fine, I have enough, I've got a plan, I've managed, I forgot about that, I'll make a budget, I'll pay you back, I have no idea what that is, I have no money.

Awkward romance

I like you, I like-like you, I maybe love you, I'll just stand over here, I'm at the door for the breeze, I'll be back in a minute, I'll see you later, I was busy, I ran out of money, I forgot, I misunderstood, I was too sad, I was too busy running, I became a vegetarian, have we met before?

Awkward noises

The mystery noise in the car when we go round a corner, the roof in the rain, my feet in the supermarket, what you do when you chew, that drip no one else can hear, everyone else's voice, ever.

Awkwardly ill

I'm ill, I'm tired, I'm sick, I'm googling, I'm not sure, I'm in pain, I don't know where, I'm suffering from something-only-1%-have, I can't do it, I can't go out, I'm in agony, I got better, I'm well enough to type, I'm only okay on the phone, I didn't know you were ill, I'm wondering why you haven't made tea?

Awkward everything

What? I wasn't listening, did you want something? I don't know, I was thinking about something else. I'll think about it. No, I won't forget, honest.

What?

Spotting an aspie adult

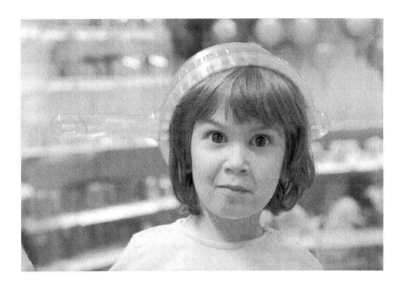

Have you ever wondered how to spot an aspie adult, at a distance, without having to get too close? It would be so convenient, wouldn't it? To be able to detect the aspieness before you are drawn in, before there is any danger of becoming part of their mad world and waking up one morning, trying to work out what happened to all your socks.

Bearing in mind there are always exceptions that prove the rule, here is what you should look for.

I often wonder if I have spotted a fellow aspie in the supermarket. Walking along the aisles, it's easier to people watch than shop, usually because I've forgotten what I need. The supermarket is a good open space where you can spot aspies as they grapple with the complex practicalities of staying alive by food shopping.

The walk

Yes, from a distance or as they pass by, the walk is a dead giveaway. It seems to veer towards extremes, either a fast paced booster effect from A to B, or a meandering wander with no visible pattern.

I'm a meanderer myself, able to get in people's way as I divert, lazily, like the Queen Mary. I drift along the aisle, knowing I need something down there, just not sure what. Deciding, as I play with the hand soap bottles, that I couldn't have needed anything important and moving on to the pizzas, totally forgetting my anti-histamines. Again.

In contrast, the go-getter aspie will leave me in their wake. They shoot past, a blur of ad hoc hair and billowing coat, the very epitome of the single-minded shopper, knowing exactly what they want and where to get it.

You might admire the determined attitude of this aspie but don't be fooled. Their pursuit of beans comes at a price. They will have a mental list and know what they want but will miss the things they forgot to put on the list or which go with what they have left at home. They will leave the store only with what was on the list and nothing else. The sense of accomplishment will fade away as they realise what they missed and they may even repeat the whole process before leaving the car park.

The attitude

This is a big one. Although not exclusively aspie, an odd attitude is also top of the list for spotters. Again, with the extremes. Your go-getter aspie, having powered through the store, will wage war at the tills (self-service only), often grumbling aloud when it goes wrong. They know it's nothing they have done, they are highly intelligent and know how to use a self-service till. And yet, like lesser mortals who have more time and a less pressing schedule (private server meet up with the Minecraft group in 20 min), they have to wait for the assistant to come and put in their code.

The shopping will be thudded onto the till, the bags will be bullied into submission; everything will be done with an air of authority that belies the fact the go-getter aspie is completely detached from what they are doing and the outwardly purposeful actions are an automatic response. This is how you behave in the shop to get in and out as quickly as possible, while your brain is utterly engrossed with a much more interesting problem.

And here I come, the meanderer, angling for my beloved self-service tills, tied to them like a love-hate relationship of Shakespearean proportions as I cling to the idea of being served without human contact, only to have them turn on me in the end.

I struggle with the bags, they seem to re-close against me. I tear them as I put my shopping in, I drop my money, forget which slot is for notes and which for coupons. I get distracted by the shoppers on the other side of the tills and forget I'm meant to be pressing the screen.

The inevitable moment comes when I'm approached by the assistant, their training having identified me as a shopper-in-need. I stand back and let them deal with whatever problem I've caused and smile distractedly, having memorised their pass-code.

Social

When there is no option but to be served at the human checkout, our two aspies stand out from the crowd in little ways. The go-getter is still on auto-pilot and could be confused with any busy person wanting to get in and out of the shop.

There are little signs the rainbow spectrum is close by: the slight twitch as they have to make eye contact with the assistant, the sudden fascination with the overhead lighting, the need to bend forward to have a look in the till, the scrutinising of the receipt as if there is something terribly wrong, holding up the queue and worrying the checkout operator, before moving off with a grunt that sounds like a satisfied bullfrog.

The meanderer, seeming so adrift as to not care, is in fact intensely impatient once in a queue. The relaxed manner around the store evaporates as soon as there is any suggestion whatsoever of A Wait. But the meanderer is good at pretending to be normal and still attempts to put on the show.

Having reached their turn in the queue, the feckless expression and worried air will mean the meanderer is probably helped with their packing without being asked. Those pesky bags will be opened and the shopping bundled in.

At this point, the stress levels rise as the shopping may be put in the *wrong* bags, in the wrong order, with too many things together. But the checkout operator is being kind in packing the bags, which means the anxiety is instantly ramped up because you can't upset them by unpacking the bags again, can you? You'll have to struggle until you get outside or re-pack it all in the back of the car.

This is where the pretending to be normal falters, pushed aside by the anxiety of the bags or the queue behind or not being able to remember if you have coupons or if you are paying by cash or card.

The meanderer will try to keep up the conversation, saying whatever seems appropriate, only realising too late that one person's appropriate is another person's so-far-off-the-wall-it-might-as-well-be-the-middle-of-the-floor.

Having gathered up the unsatisfactory bags, hoping they don't break on the way to freedom, the meanderer picks up speed and exits the shop in a state of panic, vowing never, ever to be served by a human being again.

Outside, sitting in the cars, both types of aspie come together in a common goal. Whereas other shoppers pack quickly, jump in and leave, the aspies sit behind the wheel, glowering at the receipt, sure they missed something or overpaid. Positive that they'll have to go back in and run the gauntlet of customer service.

Go-getter or meanderer, at this stage they are both plagued by the idea that the trip to the supermarket could have been so much more efficient if only they had planned better before going in. Next time it will be different. The next time will be when they stream through the shop like they are meant to be there, with a trolley no less, filling it like other people do with a week's worth of shopping.

The aspies believe next time it won't matter that they can't bear to be in the shop long enough to do a week's worth of shopping or that they are so used to using a basket they won't know how to fill a trolley. They forget that the best of lists relies on the person fulfilling it and not the act of writing it in the first place.

Relieved that next time will be a brilliant success, both aspies drive happily away, once more focused on the whole of life, all ahead and involving small things, glad to leave behind the mundanity of the tortuous supermarket, full of tricks and dangers and never twice the same.

How to talk to non-aspies: 2

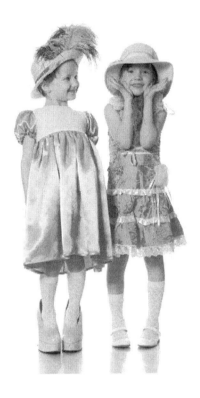

There are many ways to try talking to your non-aspie but only some of them work. Here is a short guide to what non-aspies say and what they mean. The specifics might change but the general meanings are much the same.

Once you become more familiar with the language of the non-aspie you will learn to anticipate what they are going to say and also what they mean, when in the past none of it made sense to you. After reading this you can look forward to the happiness of almost complete understanding and far less time spent trying to work out what your best beloved is trying to tell you.

Verbal Communication

Most non-aspies like to use words but they often use them in the wrong way. Here are some standard phrases which are often misused by non-aspies.

I want to talk to you

This is never good. Your non-aspie actually wants to ask you questions and receive fulsome answers. You have either done something wrong, failed to do something right or they want to talk about your feelings. Or your goldfish has died.

Why won't you talk to me?

This is often said after you have had full conversations with your non-aspie and is particularly confusing – how many words does one person need?

What they really mean is 'Why won't you talk to me about'?' and then you fill in the blank of whatever is bothering them. Usually this is used as a way to make the aspie to blame for the non-aspie explaining themselves badly or avoiding full honesty.

Unless you want to end up talking about feelings, avoid this conversation.

I should have known!

Variations on this follow some misdemeanour and suggest the non-aspie has psychic powers and so should have known you would let them down/be responsible/have avoided something important/fed the dog all the leftovers that were meant for tea (or insert appropriate domestic event).

This phrase does not invite any comment and is a sure sign no comment should be forthcoming. Strangely, it is one of those phrases which lights an aspie's indignant fire and is prone to be the start of either an argument or a storming out, or both.

You never told me!

Again with the accusations, this is for those occasions when something has occurred without proper planning, such as a doctor's appointment happening without you there or other similar important event which requires time out of the day. By not telling your non-aspie, you have created trouble or embarrassment and are in the wrong.

If you have told your best beloved and they have forgotten and you can remember the exact circumstances of this disclosure, do enlighten them even if they don't seem very receptive. Later, when you are being accused of something else, you can use this occasion as an example of how your non-aspie is also fallible and that they might have forgotten you telling them this time too.

If you remember not telling them the important thing, be ashamed, be repentant and do small jobs around the house until your non-aspie has stopped making those funny noises they find so comforting in times of stress. Do not break anything while you do the small jobs and don't recycle what looks like a pile of rubbish magazines that no one in their right mind would buy.

Are you ready yet?

The correct answer every single time is 'almost', no matter if you are naked and finishing the 14th level of Danger Dogs. The absolute wrong answer is 'ready for what?' This answer leads to unnecessary drama and fault-finding.

Where is my...?

Insert vital component of non-aspie's life which you had last – and lost. Do not admit to losing it, unless you know for certain it went in last week's bin collection or out of the car on the way onto the main road. And do not, ever, forget what the thing is as if you never laid eyes on it before.

What you should do is help look for it and seem keen to find it. This negates some of the animosity, especially as you might actually find it.

Call your mother

Insert appropriate relative/health professional/financial consultant/employer/call centre and any other phone calls you are likely to have avoided making or expected your best beloved to have made for you.

Oddly, the non-aspie does mean what they say here – they do want you to call the named person. Of course there is always more to it. What they also mean is 'call them instead of me doing it,' or 'make yourself useful for once'. By the time you are being pushed to make this type of call you have built up some resentment in your non-aspie and they are on the verge of being in a mood about it.

They will check you made the call so just get on with it.

Have you done it yet?

No, planning the call does not count.

How do you feel?

The standard response is 'fine' or similar. If your non-aspie is wanting to know how you feel about a specific event in your life then they should ask. If they want to know how you feel so they can then go on to talk about how they feel, they should say so.

All conversations involving emotions should be avoided unless you really need to talk about them and even then you can often get away with pulling faces. Your non-aspie's entreaties to know more should be treated with caution as the truth often hurts and the full, unblemished opening up of your aspie heart is probably too much for most people.

Try saying, 'I feel happy today, I hope you are too' and then find an excuse to leave quickly, in case they are not happy and want to talk about it. Return later with cake.

Non-verbal communication

Your guess is as good as mine here but there are a few things I have learned.

Shrugs

To non-aspies, shrugging seems to mean they can't be bothered to express themselves or they are bored. It is one of those actions we are meant to understand. If it is used as an answer to a question, ask again. I don't agree with allowing the shrug unless it gives you a viable excuse to avoid an awkward conversation.

Hugs

This is a tricky one as most of the time it means the non-aspie wants affection to be returned. They are rarely content with you standing there like a plinth while they do all the work. A hug is meant to be two-way and they do expect a response *every time*.

If in doubt, dodge and if there is no escape, pat them on the back slightly more softly than when the dog has done a good thing. Patting them any harder seems to feel like aggression to them and no pat at all means you have to use your arms to hug them back.

Smiles

I have no idea if most smiles are friendly or aggressive but they do seem to hide a lot of negative feelings considering the number of times enemies smile at one another. It seems to be unacceptable to grimace or glare at your enemies, even if you have spent the last ten years denigrating them to anyone who will listen. We are civilised human beings so we smile. At least, non-aspies do.

I suggest smiling back if you feel like it but it might be worth asking people if they are really happy to see you or if they smile at everyone they meet. This should sort the true friends from the rest of the world.

Holding hands

If your non-aspie is a child, you can hold their hand as they cross the road or on the way to the playground. Children need to be kept safe and hand holding is very useful for this.

If your non-aspie is an adult and they want to hold your hand, try it and see how it feels. If it immediately repulses you or they grip too hard, don't be afraid to wriggle your hand away and shake it dramatically in the air between you. Be sure to explain that you like the non-aspie but you don't want to hold hands.

A holding-hands refusal is seen as rejection, so you need to be clear. If you don't actually like the non-aspie then acting as if their hand holding physically repels you is a good way to let them know.

Eye rolling

Get used to it. This signifies those many times when your non-aspie is thinking thoughts they would rather not voice.

Face pulling

Usually the preserve of the aspie, face pulling means more when used by the non-aspie as they have to think before doing it. Consider the immediate situation and if the face pulling does not seem to fit, ask if they have a tummy ache.

Door slamming

This is done with the express intention of letting you know they aren't pleased about something (usually you are to blame for the something). You might know what is causing it, or you might be innocent of their fury; either way, avoid conflict by pretending they left the room normally and put the kettle on so it's ready for when they have calmed down.

Don't ask when tea will be ready.

An aspie's mini-guide to other people

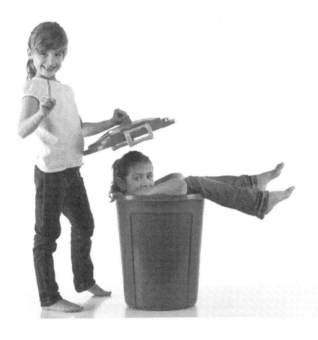

I've put together a little guide on how to react in social minefields. It's by no means all inclusive but it might help you in the future. All learned by the kind of experience which only seems funny after the event - or right in the middle of the event, if it's highly inappropriate to laugh. And to help even more, I've given you a choice of behaviours so don't feel there is only one wrong way to do things.

The Elderly

When Aunt Agatha tells you about her bad knees/aching feet/dodgy hip this is not the time to explain the effect of extra weight on the aging body or to expand into an informational discourse on obesity in modern society.

a. Smile in what you hope is a sympathetic manner and make kind noises (remember they shouldn't be the same noises you make when the dog has hurt his foot).

b. Say how sorry you are and try massaging the affected part of her body. This has the advantage of helping people discover they have more mobility than they first thought.

c. Tell Aunt Agatha that thinking about physical ailments makes you physically sick, then run off to the bathroom and stay there until she leaves.

d. Refer her to your mother who is good at pretending sympathy.

Children

Your sister's obnoxious child is ripping leaves off your potted palm and has locked the cat in the fridge again. Do not pull the child outside by the ear or tell your sister she has spawned direct from a small, dingy room in hell.

a. Tell your sister you sprayed the plant with toxic chemicals as it was infested with arachni-larvae which like feasting on tender young flesh.

b. Remove the plant and stand over the child for the remainder of the visit, giving them a fair but firm expression.

c. Ask your sister to leave as you have a terrible stomach upset and may need to change clothes (this is a last resort as sometimes family will stick around out of sympathy and then you're back to hiding in the bathroom and imitating the sounds of an embattled digestive system).

d. Refer them to your mother and go out, anywhere, until they've gone, taking the cat with you.

Friends

Your best friend comes to you with romantic problems. Do not tell her exactly where she is going wrong, how she always had bad taste in men or that if she never changes she will end up having the same crisis again and again.

a. Listen quietly and sympathetically without judging (I'm sorry, apparently this is the right approach. No, I don't understand it either).

b. Explain you have limited experience in affairs of the heart and offer to take her to your gaming club as they always need more women members there.

c. Load The Sims and show her how to manage romantic situations, including any alien encounters she might have in the future,

d. Refer her to your mother who will most likely tell her exactly where she is going wrong, remind her of her bad taste in men and then tell her to grow up, before giving her a hug.

Neighbours

Your neighbour keeps parking their car in your space or blocking your drive. Do not call the police on them to avoid direct confrontation or have a meltdown on their front step.

a. Forge a medical parking badge and put it in your car, then explain you have clients who need to see you at short notice. This should shame them into behaving but be prepared to explain what medical services you offer (IT support does not count, sorry).

b. Pay local hoodlums to hang around by their car, leering at it. Eventually they will crack and park it in a locked garage somewhere.

c. Use their car to rest against as you work on your laptop in the street, connected to their WiFi. Once you've downloaded the full series of Apoctica and her Many Admirers, you can go back inside - until the next day.

d. Stand and stare at their house at midnight, every night, until they move home (dressing in a costume is optional for this).

Work

Your work colleague outperforms you and also talks about you behind your back. They think you need to come a long way to reach their level and aren't afraid to let your boss know this. Do not, I repeat, *do not!* hack into their life online and send them into a spiral of disrepair they will never escape without professional help. (You should save this for the very special people in your life).

a. Explain to them how much you admire them and ask for their help on a regular basis. This should ensure they are so bloated with pride they end up doing your job as well as their own, thus solving the problem of your performance and freeing you up to do more important things while at work.

b. Make friends with their friends using the unusual charm you keep for emergencies, then leave them socially isolated and unhappy in the workplace.

c. Fix your boss's computer/life problems/mother's rental agreement issues and become the golden child at work, untouchable by any colleague, however talented.

d. Stare at them from across the office, wherever they are and from wherever you are, at least ten times a day. Keep your face blank and emotionless (yay for aspies!) and watch their nerves shred. When confronted, say you were thinking and didn't notice where you were looking, then temporarily stare at someone else to prove the point.

Romance

Your significant other wants to move the relationship forward. Apparently this means living together and combining all aspects of your life, like putting up with their love of soap operas and having Sunday lunch with their mother every week. Do not end the relationship on a whim or state, in a high and fraught voice, that they are allowed to use your spare room and their mother can come over as long as you are OUT.

a. Talk about your feelings (I am *so* sorry! Yes, this is what is supposed to happen! I *know*!) Be prepared to write them down first as it's easy to forget what you were going to say when you have no real intention of sharing.

b. Talk about *their* feelings and point out where they are going wrong. Once you have them crying in the middle of the rug, explain how to fix things and bask in the glow of having used logic appropriately and also avoided their mother ever visiting you again.

c. Introduce them to anime/sci-fi/Game of Thrones/Discovery Channel and make them watch everything you love. No getting out of it. Keep it up until they can't remember ever watching anything else. Then wait to see if they discuss moving in again.

d. Don't keep the cats out when they come round (I realise this is very specific advice but it can also be applied to your dog or dogs, the neighbour's small children, your embarrassing family members or a hired troupe of circus artistes).

e. Consider explaining the next stage to you is updating your relationship status to 'It's Complicated' on Facebook.

If all else fails and your significant other is still determined to make it work, consider the unusual possibility that you have found someone worth hanging onto. This is a strange concept but one that does happen to real people quite often.

However, if they still won't watch Webs of Hunger with you and still, still, *still* don't know the names of the main characters in Lord of the Rings, do consider whether you would be better off rehoming a rescue dog.

You might also like

Amanda J Harrington

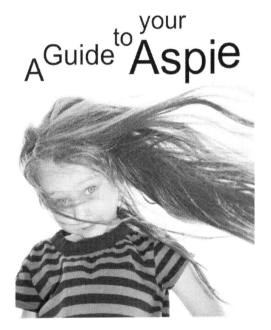

A Guide to your Aspie

Or visit the blog behind the books!

http://aspie-girl.blogspot.co.uk/

For more books and creative writing courses visit

http://www.amandajharrington.co.uk/

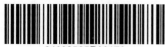

24603585R00172

Printed in Great Britain
by Amazon